Juan Augusto Hernández-Rivera
Arturo César García-Casillas
Omar Francisco Prado-Rebolledo

Reproductive responses of Charolais cattle under tropical conditions.

Juan Augusto Hernández-Rivera
Arturo César García-Casillas
Omar Francisco Prado-Rebolledo

Reproductive responses of Charolais cattle under tropical conditions.

Oestrus synchronization and fixed-time artificial insemination protocol

ScienciaScripts

Imprint
Any brand names and product names mentioned in this book are subject to trademark, brand or patent protection and are trademarks or registered trademarks of their respective holders. The use of brand names, product names, common names, trade names, product descriptions etc. even without a particular marking in this work is in no way to be construed to mean that such names may be regarded as unrestricted in respect of trademark and brand protection legislation and could thus be used by anyone.

Cover image: www.ingimage.com

This book is a translation from the original published under ISBN 978-613-9-04081-0.

Publisher:
Sciencia Scripts
is a trademark of
Dodo Books Indian Ocean Ltd. and OmniScriptum S.R.L publishing group

120 High Road, East Finchley, London, N2 9ED, United Kingdom
Str. Armeneasca 28/1, office 1, Chisinau MD-2012, Republic of Moldova, Europe
Printed at: see last page
ISBN: 978-620-8-19977-7

SUMMARY

Reproductive responses of Charolais cattle under tropical conditions.

In order to evaluate the effect of season on the reproductive responses of Charolais cows subjected to estrus synchronization protocol and fixed-time artificial insemination (**FTAI**) under tropical conditions, 48 cows were selected and randomly distributed to one of two seasons of the year, fall (n=26) and spring (n=22). The study lasted 140 days, divided into 2 periods of 70 d/season. The selection criteria were body condition, days in milk and number of calvings. During both periods the cows were under an extensive system and the same feeding regime based on pasture grass and Tanzania, and were supplemented with mineral stone and water ad libitum. The estrus synchronization protocol lasted 10 d, where: day 0 a bovine intravaginal device (**BID**) impregnated with progesterone (0.6 g) was applied and estradiol benzoate (2 mg/mL IM) was administered. On day 7 the DIB was removed and cloprostenol (0.150 mg/mL IM), estradiol cypionate (0.5 mg/mL IM), equine chorionic gonadotropin (400 IU/mL IM) were administered. IATF was performed on day 10. Ambient temperature (**TA**) and relative humidity (**RH**) data were collected every 15 min daily in each season and with these values the temperature-humidity index (**TIH**) was constructed. During autumn, the average high and low values of maximum ITH were 84 and 81 units, respectively, while in spring they were 84 and 79 units, respectively. The most critical hours of the day were from 09:00-16:00 h, reaching 85 and 87 ITH units for fall and spring, respectively. The conception rate and estrous expression tended *(P<0.10)* to improve in autumn, with respect to spring. Finally, both seasons can seriously compromise the reproductive parameters of Charolais cows under fixed-time artificial insemination in the tropics.

Key words: caloric stress, beef cattle, conception rate, artificial insemination, tropics.

ACRONYMS AND ABBREVIATIONS REFERENCE

FTAI: Fixed-Time Artificial Insemination.

AI: Artificial Insemination.

TA: Ambient Temperature.

RH: Relative Humidity.

ITH: Temperature-humidity index.

EC: Caloric stress.

mHa: Millions of hectares.

kg: Kilograms.

cm: Centimeters.

GnRH: Gonadotropin-releasing hormone.

FSH: Follicle Stimulating Hormone.

LH: Luteinizing Hormone.

PGF2α: Prostaglandin F2α.

E_2 : Estrogen.

P_4 : Progesterone.

DIB: Progesterone impregnated bovine intravaginal device.

DBS: Estradiol cypionate.

eCG: Equine chorionic gonadotropin.

IM: Intramuscular.

THEMATIC CONTENT

I. INTRODUCTION

Performing reproductive service at the most appropriate time can be a great challenge (Espinoza-Villavicencio et al., 2021), especially when heat stress decreases the proportion of embryos that become blastocysts (Verdoljak et al., 2018) and in autumn the peak of pasture production is taken advantage of to get more cows pregnant (Espinoza-Villavicencio et al., 2021). Reproductive indexes of cattle in tropical regions are poor, their pregnancy percentages are managed from 45-55%, with calving intervals of 18 months (Verdoljak et al., 2018). The best reproductive performance in dual-purpose cattle is obtained in dry and rainy seasons (Loyo et al., 2018); however, on hot days and unavailable shade from trees usually produce losses of newborn calves.

Artificial insemination (**AI**) is a tool used for genetic improvement of livestock in the tropics (Riveros et al., 2018). Fixed-time artificial insemination (**FTAI**) is a reproductive technique that has had great development (Pérez et al., 2015). This type of protocol is used as the best alternative for ovulation and fertilization control. Reproductive efficiency is an important aspect in bovine production, which has a cost-benefit impact on bovine production (Pérez et al., 2015). The use of this type of alternative increases the number of cows inseminated in a short period of time (Avalos et al., 2018). The use of IATF protocols based on previous studies show that the pregnancy percentage is 40-50 % (Espinoza-Villavicencio et al., 2021). To consider that IATF was successful, the highest number of pregnant cows and birth of live calves in fixed time should be obtained (Avalos et al., 2018). The benefits of IATF is the reduction of insemination time, short postpartum period and improved results of cows with calves at foot (Aro and Alvarez, 2019). The most important limiting factor of this protocol is the reduction of fertility after induced estrus (Parra et al., 2017). The low levels of postpartum pregnancy are due to the fact that cattle producers continue to use traditional methods of reproduction (Perez et al., 2022).

IATF increases the pregnancy rate of herds without waiting for heat detection (Horrach et al., 2021). Beef herds develop reproductive management plans to optimize the productivity time of beef cattle (Pérez et al., 2022). With the application of reproductive biotechnologies, it is possible to choose the best time to carry out matings according to the protocol used (Pérez et al., 2022). Therefore, the objective of this study was to evaluate the effect of time of year (spring and fall) on the conception rate of Charolais beef cows subjected to an estrus synchronization protocol and fixed-time artificial insemination under tropical conditions.

II. LITERATURE REVIEW

2.1 Cattle raising in Mexico

In livestock production in Mexico, the purpose is to produce good quality food, which is accessible to society in general (Rojas et al., 2021). Cattle ranching in rural environments is the most important activity, since it allows the practice of it in adverse climatic conditions (Puebla et al., 2018). There are different production systems in cattle ranching, ranging from technified systems to backyard systems (Granados et al., 2018). These systems are developed in Mexico according to the availability of natural resources in the country (Parra and Magaña, 2019), where traditional systems are the most developed (Granados et al., 2018). The production system in the dry tropics is cow-calf, pasture development, fattening on pasture and feedlot, for the humid tropics, cow-calf (dual purpose), fattening on pasture and feedlot systems are managed (Gutiérrez et al., 2005).

Mexico allocates 145 million hectares (73% of the national territory) for agricultural activities (FAO, 2017), where 58% of the surface is destined for cattle grazing. In 2021, the national bovine inventory was concentrated in 71, 997, 770 head of cattle, of which the states with the highest national production of beef were: Veracruz, Jalisco, Chiapas, Chihuahua and Michoacán; the states with the highest milk production: Jalisco, Durango, Chihuahua, Coahuila and Guanajuato; the states with the highest dual-purpose cattle production: Veracruz, Jalisco, Chiapas, Chihuahua and Michoacán (**Figure 1**). The development of livestock activities is carried out throughout the Mexican territory; however, the tropical region stands out for concentrating 33% of the total existing cattle population at the national level (SIAP, 2018).

Mexico imports a considerable amount of beef from the United States (81%) and Canada (18%) for domestic consumption, at the same time, it exports 85% of the almost 2 million tons produced per year to four predominant destinations: United States (61%), Japan (26%), Russia (7%) and Korea (5%) (Jiménez and Sánchez, 2014). However, in Mexico beef consumption is on the decline (Puebla et al., 2018), in 2000 more than 22 kilograms of beef were consumed per person, thus decreasing to 14.8 kilograms of beef in 2016 (FIRA, 2017).

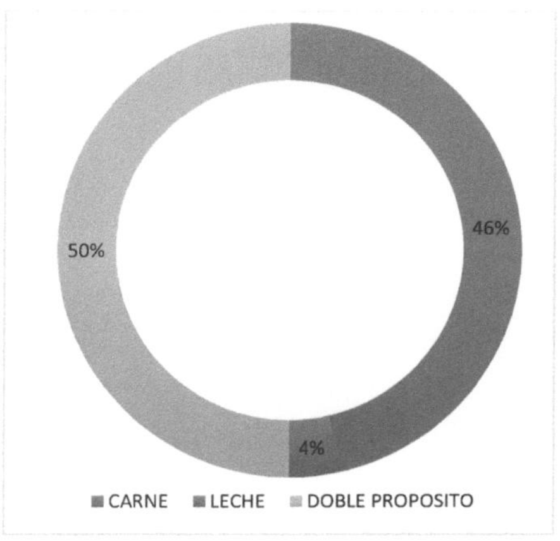

Figure 1. Cattle production in Mexico.

Prepared from SIAP (2022).

2.2 Cattle raising in the state of Colima

The state of Colima has an area of 545.5 thousand hectares representing 0.30% of the national surface, of which 41.8 thousand hectares are used as pasture for livestock use (INEGI, 2020).

The main base for cattle ranching is native grasslands or natural pastures. Cattle ranching in the state of Colima covers 67% of the state's total surface area (**Figure 2**). In the northern zone of the state, dual-purpose cattle are grouped together, with 13% of production; in the central zone, beef cattle predominate with 37%; in the coastal zone, beef cattle and, to a lesser extent, dual-purpose cattle are found. In the northern zone of the state, the predominant breeds are Zebu crossed with American Swiss and European Swiss, Limousin and Simbra; in the central zone, production systems are based on guinea grass pastures, African star, llanero and native species; in the coastal zone, the extensive system with native grasses predominates in low deciduous forest pastures, fattening and dual purpose in cultivated pastures under palm trees. (SIAP, 2022).

For the year 2021, the beef cattle inventory was 181,572 head, for dairy cattle it was 8,239 head and 189,811 head of dual-purpose cattle (SIAP, 2022).

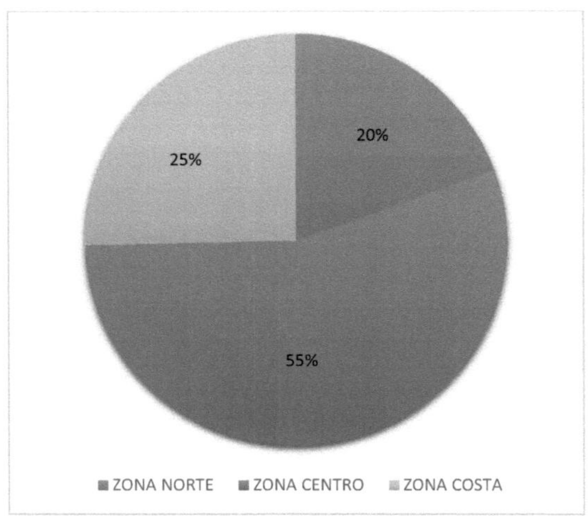

Figure 2. Cattle production by zone in the state of Colima.

Prepared from SIAP (2022).

2.3 Characteristics of the Charolais breed

The Charolais breed originated in the central western and southwestern regions of France, in the provinces of Charolles and Niemen (FAO, 1968). It is a meat-producing breed, with abundant musculature in the hindquarters, where cuts of higher meat quality are obtained. These cattle reach a high weight in adulthood, with males weighing from 1000 to 1400 kg and females from 750 to 900 kg (Utrera et al., 2021). They are large and heavy cattle, white or cream colored, the skin is loose and of medium thickness; the hair is soft, of medium length and sometimes has a woolly appearance, the head is short, deep and wide, the eyes are dark and the horns are pale (Utrera et al., 2007).

Males have a pronounced muscular thickening in the cervical region and have a long and deep body, the pelvis is of moderate length and slope, the limbs are quite long and with strong bones (**Table 1**).

Table 1. Live weight and zoometric averages of Charolais cattle.

	MALES		FEMALES	
	1 YEAR	**ADULTS**	**2 YEARS**	**ADULTS**
Live weight (kg)	516	1086	614	812
Height at withers (cm)	122	142	130	137
Chest circumference (cm)	182	239	199	217
Thoracic depth (cm)	46	64	51	59
Croup width (cm)	44	55	53	57

Adapted from FAO (1968).

It is one of the most important cattle breeds in Mexico, due to its productivity in meat production and is found in tropical, subtropical, temperate and arid climate regions (Utrera et al., 2007).

2.4 Caloric stress, EC

CE can be defined as the action of stimuli that are provoked by the environment or other factors (Marcoppido et al., 2018), affecting the physiological systems of animals such as the nervous, endocrine, circulatory, digestive, reproductive, etc. (de Aguiar et al., 2020). CE refers to the combination of factors that can cause an elevation in body temperature (Becker et al., 2020).

The effects of CE can be of two types:

1. Direct: alterations in metabolism to adapt to increased heat and hormonal repercussions (Pires et al., 2021).
2. Indirect: alteration of feed quality and quantity, breed, physiological state, milk production level, age, skin color, exposure to the environment and animal variation (Pires et al., 2021).

On the other hand, CE can be classified as mild, moderate and severe (**Figure 3**), again, depending on the temperature and/or humidity in different beef or dairy cattle production systems. Animal thermoregulation is a neuroendocrine mechanism, which is achieved by physiological and behavioral mechanisms (Pires et al., 2021). Temperature is the main factor in CE and is associated with humidity and solar radiation. Additionally, CE can be generated by oscillation at high temperatures or combination of negative factors in a short period of time (Armstrong, 1994).

The temperature of the environment considerably affects the animal's body temperature, increasing its metabolism by 10% (Marcoppido et al., 2018). Due to the physiological changes that occur in animals, the reproductive part has been affected, due to the detection of estrus in high temperatures becomes more complicated (Correa et al., 2016).

The species with the highest productivity in the field is *Bos taurus* cattle, however, *Bos indicus* cattle despite being able to withstand more CD than European breeds, their physical conditions in the tropics lead them to suffer CD as well, which affects their productivity (Fournel et al., 2017). The environmental temperature ranges reported as comfort in *Bos indicus* animals are usually wider than in *Bos taurus, which* range from 0 to 20 °C, with 70% environmental humidity (Pires et al., 2021). Being under tropical conditions, the main problem for cattle is a drop in production, in addition to the fact that CE generates a deficiency in heat dissipation mechanisms (Mbuthia et al., 2021).

Low fertility during the summer is associated with the warm months (June-September), which negatively impacts fertility in the fall months (October-November) (Wolfenson et al., 2000). It is a fairly common condition to manage for animal welfare as it is related to the regulation of the follicular phase of the estrous cycle and ovulation (Fournel et al., 2017). It impacts the reproductive axis of the hypothalamus by affecting GnRH secretion, and the pituitary gland by affecting gonadotropin secretion (Regalado and Alvarez, 2020), in addition to being related to decreased conception rates (Thatcher et al., 1994), because it affects follicular dynamics, corpus luteum development, luteal P_4 production and embryonic development (Ronchi et al., 2001).

There are some methods to decrease the EC such as the provision of shade, unrestricted supply of quality water, deep beds, cooling systems based on fans and sprinklers, others based on air turbines in combination with water, etc. (Mbuthia et al., 2021).

2.5 Reproductive physiology

Female cattle are considered to be annual polyestrians. The estrous cycle can be defined as the biological reproductive cycle of females, where estrus and ovulation occur (Ronchi et al., 2001). It is a period comprising two consecutive estrus, in which recurring events occur and is divided into different phases (Hernández, 2012), the luteal phase and the follicular phase (Ronchi et al., 2001). Behavioral, morphophysiological, histological and biochemical changes of the genital tract occur, which allows the acceptance of the male for mating. Hernandez (2012) mentions that the duration of the estrous cycle ranges from 17 to 23 days, with an average of 21 days. In heifers, the estrous cycle occurs at puberty (6-12 months of age) (Ronchi et al., 2001).

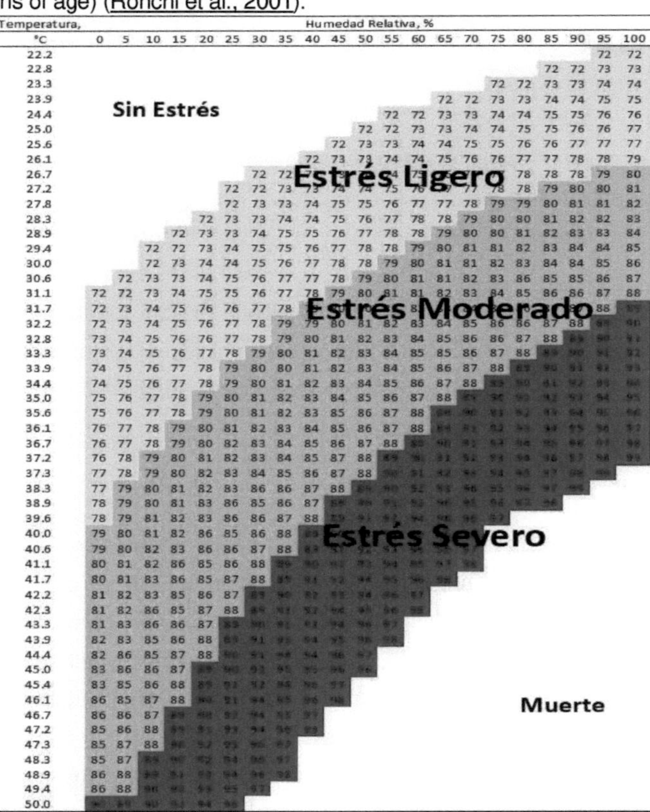

Temperatura,	Humedad Relativa, %																				
°C	0	5	10	15	20	25	30	35	40	45	50	55	60	65	70	75	80	85	90	95	100
22.2																				72	72
22.8																		72	72	73	73
23.3																72	72	73	73	74	74
23.9														72	72	73	73	74	74	75	75
24.4												72	72	73	73	74	74	75	75	76	76
25.0											72	72	73	73	74	74	75	75	76	76	77
25.6										72	73	73	74	74	75	75	76	76	77	77	77
26.1									72	73	73	74	74	75	76	76	77	77	78	78	79
26.7							72	72	[illegible]	[illegible]	[illegible]	[illegible]	[illegible]	[illegible]	[illegible]	[illegible]	78	78	78	79	80
27.2						72	72	73	73	74	74	75	76	[illegible]	77	78	78	79	80	80	81
27.8						72	73	73	74	75	75	76	77	77	78	79	79	80	81	81	82
28.3					72	73	73	74	74	75	76	77	78	78	79	80	80	81	82	82	83
28.9				72	73	73	74	75	75	76	77	78	78	79	80	80	81	82	83	83	84
29.4			72	72	73	74	75	75	76	77	78	78	79	80	81	81	82	83	84	84	85
30.0			72	73	74	74	75	76	77	78	78	79	80	81	81	82	83	84	84	85	86
30.6		72	73	73	74	75	76	77	77	78	79	80	81	81	82	83	86	85	85	86	87
31.1	72	72	73	74	75	75	76	77	78	79	80	81	81	82	83	84	85	86	86	87	88
31.7	72	73	74	75	76	76	77	78	[illegible]	[illegible]	[illegible]	[illegible]	[illegible]	[illegible]	[illegible]	[illegible]	[illegible]	[illegible]	[illegible]	88	[illegible]
32.2	72	73	74	75	76	77	78	79	79	80	81	82	83	84	85	86	86	87	88	[illegible]	[illegible]
32.8	73	74	75	76	76	77	78	79	80	81	82	83	84	85	86	86	87	88	[illegible]	[illegible]	[illegible]
33.3	73	74	75	76	77	78	79	80	81	82	83	84	85	85	86	87	88	[illegible]	[illegible]	[illegible]	[illegible]
33.9	74	75	76	77	78	79	80	80	81	82	83	84	85	86	87	88	[illegible]	[illegible]	[illegible]	[illegible]	[illegible]
34.4	74	75	76	77	78	79	80	81	82	83	84	85	86	87	88	[illegible]	[illegible]	[illegible]	[illegible]	[illegible]	[illegible]
35.0	75	76	77	78	79	80	81	82	83	84	85	86	87	88	[illegible]	[illegible]	[illegible]	[illegible]	[illegible]	[illegible]	[illegible]
35.6	75	76	77	78	79	80	81	82	83	85	86	87	88	[illegible]	[illegible]	[illegible]	[illegible]	[illegible]	[illegible]	[illegible]	[illegible]
36.1	76	77	78	79	80	81	82	83	84	85	86	87	88	[illegible]	[illegible]	[illegible]	[illegible]	[illegible]	[illegible]	[illegible]	[illegible]
36.7	76	77	78	79	80	82	83	84	85	86	87	88	[illegible]	[illegible]	[illegible]	[illegible]	[illegible]	[illegible]	[illegible]	[illegible]	[illegible]
37.2	76	78	79	80	81	82	83	84	85	87	88	[illegible]	[illegible]	[illegible]	[illegible]	[illegible]	[illegible]	[illegible]	[illegible]	[illegible]	[illegible]
37.3	77	78	79	80	82	83	84	85	86	87	88	[illegible]	[illegible]	[illegible]	[illegible]	[illegible]	[illegible]	[illegible]	[illegible]	[illegible]	
38.3	77	79	80	81	82	83	86	86	87	88	[illegible]	[illegible]	[illegible]	[illegible]	[illegible]	[illegible]	[illegible]	[illegible]	[illegible]		
38.9	78	79	80	81	83	86	85	86	87	[illegible]	[illegible]	[illegible]	[illegible]	[illegible]	[illegible]	[illegible]	[illegible]	[illegible]			
39.6	78	79	81	82	83	86	86	87	88	[illegible]	[illegible]	[illegible]	[illegible]	[illegible]	[illegible]	[illegible]					
40.0	79	80	81	82	86	85	86	88	[illegible]	[illegible]	[illegible]	[illegible]	[illegible]	[illegible]	[illegible]						
40.6	79	80	82	83	86	86	87	88	[illegible]	[illegible]	[illegible]	[illegible]	[illegible]	[illegible]	[illegible]						
41.1	80	81	82	86	85	86	88	[illegible]	[illegible]	[illegible]	[illegible]	[illegible]	[illegible]	[illegible]	[illegible]						
41.7	80	81	83	86	85	87	88	[illegible]	[illegible]	[illegible]	[illegible]	[illegible]	[illegible]	[illegible]							
42.2	81	82	83	85	86	87	[illegible]	[illegible]	[illegible]	[illegible]	[illegible]	[illegible]	[illegible]								
42.3	81	82	86	85	87	88	[illegible]	[illegible]	[illegible]	[illegible]	[illegible]	[illegible]	[illegible]								
43.3	81	83	86	86	87	[illegible]	[illegible]	[illegible]	[illegible]	[illegible]	[illegible]	[illegible]									
43.9	82	83	85	86	88	[illegible]	[illegible]	[illegible]	[illegible]	[illegible]	[illegible]	[illegible]									
44.4	82	86	85	87	88	[illegible]	[illegible]	[illegible]	[illegible]	[illegible]	[illegible]										
45.0	83	86	86	87	[illegible]	[illegible]	[illegible]	[illegible]	[illegible]	[illegible]	[illegible]										
45.4	83	85	86	88	[illegible]	[illegible]	[illegible]	[illegible]	[illegible]	[illegible]											
46.1	86	85	87	88	[illegible]	[illegible]	[illegible]	[illegible]	[illegible]	[illegible]											
46.7	86	86	87	[illegible]	[illegible]	[illegible]	[illegible]	[illegible]	[illegible]												
47.2	85	86	88	[illegible]	[illegible]	[illegible]	[illegible]	[illegible]	[illegible]												
47.3	85	87	88	[illegible]	[illegible]	[illegible]	[illegible]	[illegible]													
48.3	85	87	[illegible]	[illegible]	[illegible]	[illegible]	[illegible]	[illegible]													
48.9	86	88	[illegible]	[illegible]	[illegible]	[illegible]	[illegible]	[illegible]													
49.4	86	88	[illegible]	[illegible]	[illegible]	[illegible]	[illegible]														
50.0	[illegible]	[illegible]	[illegible]	[illegible]	[illegible]	[illegible]															

Sin Estrés
Estrés Ligero
Estrés Moderado
Estrés Severo
Muerte

Figure 3. Temperature and humidity index (TIH). Calculated from ambient temperature (TA, ºC) and relative humidity (RH, %). Yellow= light. Orange: moderate. Red: severe.

Retrieved from Wiersma (1990).

On the other hand, proestrus has an average duration of 2 to 3 days, characterized by the absence of a functional corpus luteum and maturation of the ovulatory follicle (Hernandez, 2012). FSH induces rapid growth of a dominant ovarian follicle that elevates estrogen concentration (Ronchi et al., 2001). There is a decrease in plasma P_4 levels that results in the release of PGF2α from the endometrium and precedes estrus. Close to estrus, the preovulatory follicle grows in size and produces high amounts of estradiol (Sheldon et al., 2006).

During the estrous phase, luteinizing hormone (LH) levels increase in response to the estrogen elevation (Ronchi et al., 2001), the female becomes receptive to the male and allows copulation. A dominant follicle is found which elevates estradiol and inhibin concentrations in the follicular fluid.

Likewise, during metaestrus, ovulation occurs with the rupture of the dominant follicle and the release of the gamete. A new corpus luteum develops where serum P_4 concentrations increase to levels greater than 1 ng/mL (Ronchi et al., 2001).

Finally, during diestrous, which can occur between the 5th to 7th day of the cycle (Hernández, 2012). In this phase the corpus luteum finishes its maturation process, if there is an embryo in the uterus maternal recognition signals are sent that stop the luteolysis process (Boeta et al., 2018).

2.6 Reproductive endocrinology

Hormones are chemical molecules produced in specific organs, which are released into the blood in small amounts and exert their effect on a target organ (Matamoros and Sanhueza, 2017). The control of the estrous cycle involves the interrelated secretion of several hormones that are produced in the hypothalamus, anterior pituitary, ovaries and uterus (Reece, 2015), which involves the following hormones:

Like GnRH, it is synthesized by hypothalamic neurons and secreted in a pulsatile manner in the median eminence within the hypothalamo-pituitary portal system (Colazo and Mapletoft, 2022). The secretion of GnRH from the hypothalamus to the pituitary gland via the hypothalamic portal blood system thus releases the gonadotropin hormones FSH and LH (Hafez and Hafez, 2002). FSH is responsible for the process of ovarian steroidogenesis, growth and follicular maturation (Fernandez, 2008). Meanwhile, LH receptors are increased in the granulosa cells of the dominant follicle which is sensitive to the LH surge that produces ovulation (Hafez and Hafez, 2002).

E_2 are steroidal hormones produced in the follicle, specifically in the cells of the internal theca, whose target organs are the uterus, oviducts, vagina, vulva and central nervous system, to stimulate estrus and/or receptivity of females to the male, and can also stimulate the hypothalamus by positive feedback to release GnRH (Fernandez, 2008).

P_4 is a steroid hormone produced by the corpus luteum. It prepares the uterus to receive the fertilized oocyte and favors implantation in uterine horns (Ronchi et al., 2001). It also exerts a negative feedback on the hypothalamus (Boeta et al., 2018).

PGF2α, are made of unsaturated fatty acids and are synthesized in endometrial cells (Hafez and Hafez, 2002). The release of PGF2α from the myometrium indicates regression of the corpus luteum (Hernandez, 2012). It is identified as the luteolytic, myometrial stimulating hormone, generating contractions in the smooth muscles of the uterus. PGF2α is produced in endometrial cells in the last phase of the estrous cycle when there is no embryo, in granulosa cells of the dominant follicle and in luteal cells at the end of the diestrous (Davidson and Stabenfeldt, 2014). P_4 and E_2 can directly affect the basal secretion of PGF2α by the endometrium (Ronchi et al., 2001).

On the other hand, the hypothalamus-pituitary-gonadal axis is responsible for the control of the reproductive cycle in females and males (**Figure 4**), which fulfills two main functions: the synthesis of steroid hormones (steroidogenesis) and the production of gametes (gametogenesis; Hafez and Hafez, 2002). The hypothalamus is the nervous center responsible for coordinating a large number of activities in the organism (Ramirez and Lilido, 2006). The pituitary gland, also known as the hypophysis, is located in a depression in the superior aspect of the sphenoid bone (Hernández, 2012). It is made up of two parts: the adenohypophysis, which is responsible for the production of gonadotropins, and the neurohypophysis, which is responsible for storing antidiuretic hormone and oxytocin (Fernández, 2008).

It all starts with the pulsatile secretion of GnRH hormone from parvocellular neurosecretory neurons, periventricular nucleus, paraventricular and preoptic area of the hypothalamus (Gomez et al., 2014). The action of FSH and LH hormone is essential for the development of antral follicles (Hafez and Hafez, 2002). The preovulatory LH peak generates luteinization of the granulosa cells of the preovarian follicle and begins to generate P_4 (Van der Hurk and Zhao, 2005).

In mammals, the acquisition of secondary sexual characteristics, reproductive function and aging are regulated by the effect of the hypothalamic-pituitary-gonadal (HPG) axis (Hernández, 2012). In males, LH and FSH hormones activate testicular sex steroid production and spermatogenesis (Hernandez, 2012).

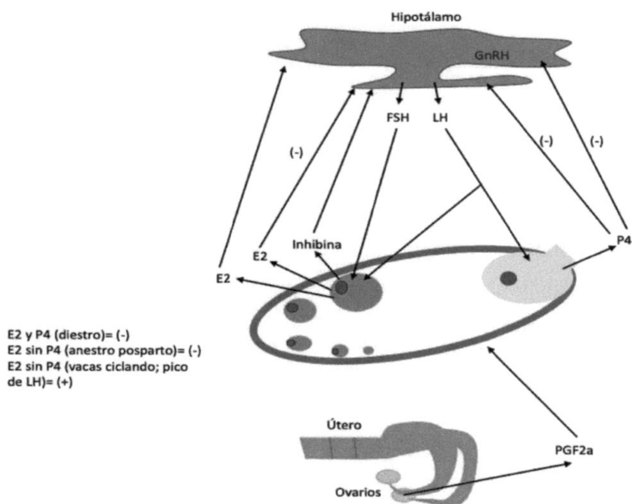

Figure 4. Feedback between hypothalamus, pituitary and ovaries.

Adapted from Hernández (2012).

2.7 Reproductive parameters

Puberty is considered to be reached when the animal produces viable gametes for fertilization for the first time (Bartolomé, 2009); in the case of females, it is when the first ovulation occurs and the first estrus is manifested. Heifers reach puberty at 17 months of age with variations of 12-21 months (**Table 2**).

Hernández, 2012, indicated that the age of heifers has a close relationship with the weight and size of the animal so that they can be ready for service to avoid abnormal calving. Female cattle can be served for the first time between 15 to 19 months of age, weighing 380 kg to maximize their productive performance (Norman et al., 2017).

A heifer's first calving, which depends on management and feeding during the growth period, occurs between 32 and 42 months (Hernández, 2012).
The productive life of a cow is influenced by the age at first service; cows calving at two years of age have better productive and reproductive performance (Correa et al., 2016).

Table2. Age-based reproductive parameters of cattle in tropical regions.

PARAMETERS	MONTHS
Age at puberty	17 (12-21)
Age at first service	24 (20-27)
Age at first conception	25.5 (21-29)
Age at first birth	34.7 (30-39)

Elaborated from Anta (1989).

The days between calving and first estrus in tropical conditions can be two to more months (**Table 3**; Alvarez et al., 2020).

Days from calving to first service (**DPPS**) is the time that elapses from calving to first service, ideally no more than 85 days (Ríos and Villagómez, 2020).

$$DPPS= \frac{IPC\ en\ dias}{NVP}$$

IPC: Interval childbirth - conception

NVP: Number of pregnant cows

The calving-conception interval (**CCI**) is the days open, the time in which cows remain empty. Ideally, it should not exceed 100 days (Ríos and Villagómez, 2020).

The inter-calving interval (**IEP**) is the period that elapses between a calving and a new conception (Ríos and Villagómez, 2020). The calving interval is the most widely used productive parameter as an indicator of reproductive efficiency. The first 120 days of lactation is the time when cows show the best productive performance (Risco et al., 2009), it is important to get cows pregnant before 90 days after calving.

$$IEP = \frac{Días\ entre\ parto\ y\ parto}{Total\ de\ vacas}$$

Days to service (**DS**) is the time interval between the first service and the actual service (Risco et al., 2009). The age at first conception in heifers and the interval between calving and conception in adult cows can influence SD (Severino et al., 2021).

Table 3. Reproductive parameters in tropical cows.

PARAMETERS	AVERAGE
First heat interval, d	78
First service interval, d	102
Conception delivery interval, d	149
Interval between deliveries, d	447
Services per concept, n	1.8
Mounts by conception, n	1.7
Births per reproductive life, n	3.4

Elaborated from Anta (1989).

The percentage of conception at first service (**PCPS**; **Table 4**), the percentage of conception at first service is calculated to evaluate the fertility of animals under more homogeneous conditions (Risco et al., 2009).

$$PCPS = \frac{NVP\ al\ 1\ servicio}{NVS}\ x\ 100$$

NVP: Number of pregnant cows.

NVS: Number of cows served.

Services per conception is the number of inseminations necessary for a cow to become pregnant (Palacios et al., 2022). It is considered acceptable from 1.5 to 1.8 services per conception (Kruif, 1978).

$$SPC=\frac{No.total\ de\ servicios}{NVP}$$

Fertility rate (**FFR**) is the number of cows that become pregnant during a given period (Lozano et al., 2020). The total fertility rate is 60%.

Table 4. Percentage of conception in tropical cows.

PARAMETER	%
Conception at the first service	52.1
Conception with AI	44.7
Conception with natural mating	54.2
Total fertility rate	60.4

Elaborated from Anta (1989).

2.8 Reproductive efficiency

Reproductive efficiency is the production of one calf per cow, within the biological period allowed to maximize profitability, fertility and profit increase (Cattle, 2020). Low reproductive efficiency is associated with cow or herd health (Torres et al., 2022). Loss of gestation results in an increasing number of non-pregnant cows which causes maintenance costs to accumulate (Tapia and Hepp, 2020).

Reproductive efficiency depends on factors such as nutrition, body condition, management during peripartum, individual fertility, sires, age, inbreeding percentage, bull age, month and process (Rodriguez, 2021).

Table 5. Indicators to determine reproductive efficiency in female cattle.

INDEX	RATING		
	DEFICIENT	GOOD	META
Interval between births (months)	13.5	13	12.5
Pregnancy delivery time (days)	130	100	90
Time to first service (days)	90	80	70
Services by concept	2	1.8	1.6
Age at first birth (months)	27	26	24

Elaborated from Zemjanis (1962).

2.9 Artificial Insemination

Artificial insemination (**AI**) is a technique based on the deposition of semen in the uterus of females through instruments (Giraldo et al., 2017). The objective is to deposit a determined number of live spermatozoa in the genital tract of the female and for fertilization to occur (Hafez and Hafez, 2002). AI is a means to help improve the production conditions of production units (Boeta et al., 2018). To optimize the process and increase the pregnancy rate, the ovaries must be hormonally stimulated (Perez et al. 2015), to control ovulation and approach the correct time for AI (Parra et al., 2017). Among the main success factors for AI are semen quality, suitability of protocols, etc.

Some of its advantages are the low cost of semen and its application, lower risks involved in natural mating, and the only disadvantages are that it must be carried out by trained personnel (Shipka and Ellis, 1999).

2.10 Fixed-Time Artificial Insemination

To maximize the reproductive genetic potential of cattle, it is necessary to reduce the days open in the first three months postpartum, obtaining pregnancy as soon as possible (Vallejo et al., 2017). Fixed-time artificial insemination is a technique in which hormones are used and allows synchronization of estrus and ovulations (INTAGRI, 2018). It is defined as the biotechnology for the application of semen in the genital tract of a female at the effective moment to generate fertilization (Giraldo, 2014), and thus be able to inseminate a large number of animals in a short period of time.

Ávalos et al., 2018 comments that using the IATF technique has allowed the use of genetically superior bulls to maximize the quality of the calves produced. However, in the use of this technique, its application in lactating cows is difficult due to the fact that they are together with the calf for a prolonged time (Vallejo et al., 2017).

The most commonly used IATF protocols begin with the application of IVD and estradiol benzoate on day 0, and at the end of day 7 or 8, PGF2α and estrogens (cypionate or velerate) are applied (Carvalho et al., 2008). In order to perform an IATF, a simulated estrous cycle must be performed with the application of all the hormones that allow ovulation (Fricke et al., 2016a), a batch of females that have calved between 40 to 60 days must be selected and prepared to ovulate at the same time (Fricke et al., 2016b). Finally, the stress generated by handling animals during IATF can translate into a decrease in conception rate (Correa et al., 2016).

2.11 Embryo transfer

Embryo transfer is a method of acquiring eggs from a donor female that are transferred to the reproductive tract of a recipient female (Navarro et al., 2021a). The primary objective of this technology is to maximize the number of progeny of genetically superior animals and to disseminate their germplasm worldwide (Gallegos et al., 2022). With the use of embryo transfer, more than one hundred offspring have been acquired from a cow during her reproductive life. Embryo transfer technology requires physical and pharmacological selection and management (Mapletoft, 2006).

Some of its advantages are: taking advantage of the genetic and reproductive potential of the females, exchange of international genetic value, acquiring more offspring from each embryo (Brito, 1999).

Some of its disadvantages are that the number of embryos obtained per donor is 6.5 embryos (Viana, 2019), high variability in response to hormonal treatments by bovine females (Mikkola and Taponen, 2017). A drawback of the technique is the detection of recipient estrus (Navarro et al., 2021a).

In order to obtain good results in embryo transfer programs, it depends on aspects such as the type of protocol to be used, the hormones used, the nutritional status of the animal, breed, age, climate and management (Navarro et al., 2021b).

2.12 Estrus synchronization protocols

Cows receiving a PGF2α-based treatment in the presence of a corpus luteum show estrus between 2-6 days later to receive AI (**Figure 5**) and obtain a fertility rate similar to that of natural estrus.

This protocol is applied as follows:

DAY 0: PGF2α.

Day 2-6: Heat observation and AM/PM insemination.

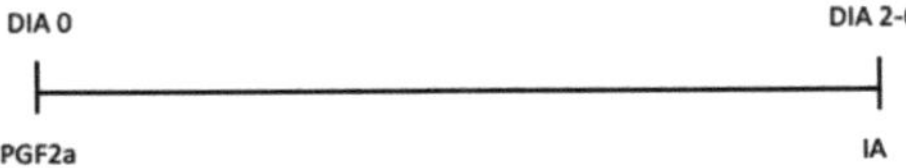

Figure 5. Oestrus synchronization protocol based on prostaglandin F2α.

Elaborated from Obando, 2020.

Another estrus synchronization protocol is Ovsynch (**Figure 6**), which is used to obtain ovulation in dairy cows, this protocol combines the hormones GnRH and PGF2α, it allows AI without detection of estrus (Gutierrez et al., 2005).

This protocol is applied as follows:

Day 0: Application of GnRH.

Day 7: PGF2α.

Day 9: Application of GnRH.

Day 10: IATF: Insemination 16 hours after the second dose of GnRH.

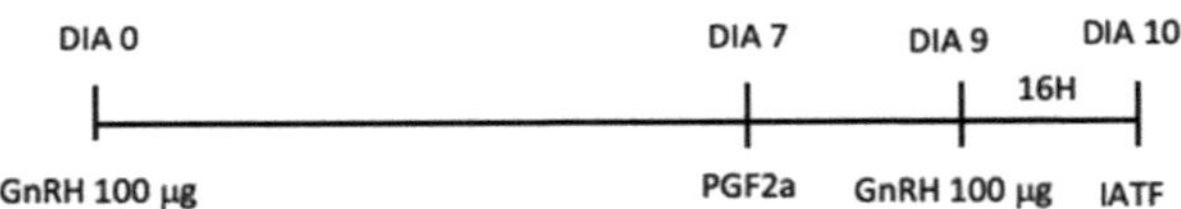

Figure 6. Ovsynch estrus synchronization protocol.

The CoSynch estrus synchronization protocol (**Figure 7**) unlike Ovsynch is that it receives IATF on the same day as the second dose of GnRH (Marizancén and Artunduaga, 2017).

This protocol is applied as follows:

Day 0: GnRH.

Day 7: PGF2α

Day 10: GnRH and IATF.

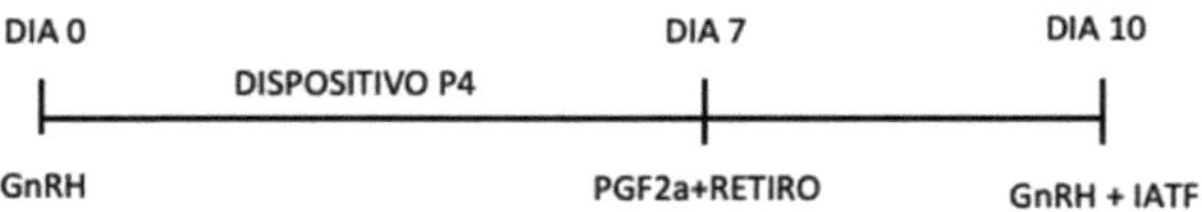

Figure 7. Cosynch synchronization protocol.

Other estrus synchronization protocols can be based on P_4 , estradiol benzoate (BE), PGF2α and IATF (**Figure 8**; Marizancén and Artunduaga, 2017).

This protocol is applied as follows:

Day 0: P device$_4$ + estradiol benzoate.

Day 7: Removal of device P_4 + PGF2α.

Day 8: BE.

Day 9 or 10: Inseminate 30 h after applying BE.

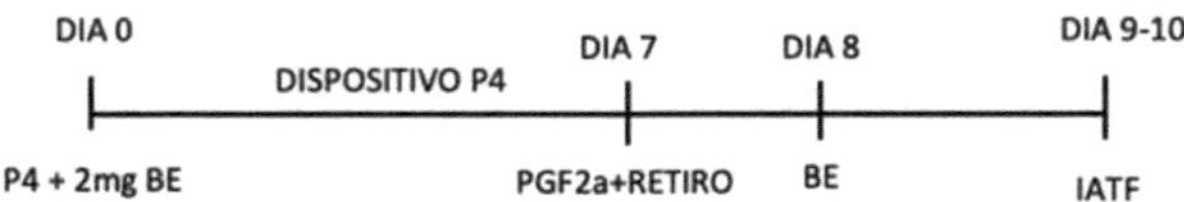

Figure 8. Estrus synchronization protocol based on progesterone, estradiol benzoate and fixed-time artificial insemination.

Other estrus synchronization protocols may use P_4 , ECP and eCG plus IATF devices (**Figure 9**).

Day 0: Device P_4 + BE.

Day 8: Removal of P device$_4$ + PGF2α + estradiol cypionate + eCG.

Day 10: Inseminate 44-48 hours after removal of the intravaginal progesterone device (Obando, 2020).

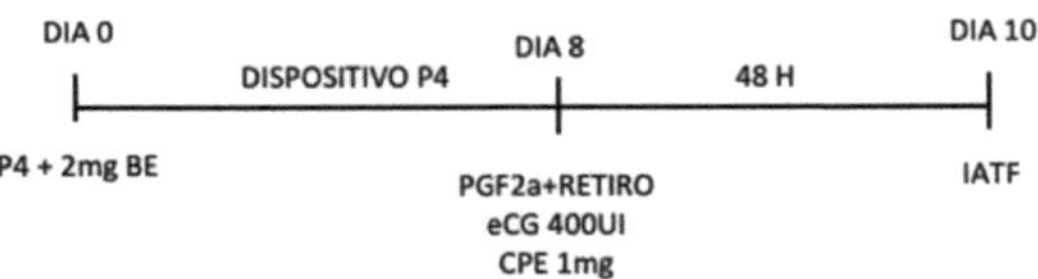

Figure 9. Estrus synchronization protocol based on progesterone, estradiol cypionate and equine chorionic gonadotropin devices.

2.13 Diagnostic methods of gestation

Early diagnosis of pregnancy is a fundamental practice for the reproductive efficiency of herds (López, 2021). The purpose of this test is the identification of animals that are not pregnant, in order to serve them again in the shortest possible time.

Rectal palpation is the most commonly used method because it is effective and inexpensive (Pohler et al., 2017). It can be performed 45 days after service, thus allowing the detection of pregnancy.

The examiner should detect at least one of these pathognomonic signs of gestation:

- Palpation of the amniotic vesicle.
- Placentomas (cotyledons and caruncles).
- Fetus.
- Prominence of the middle uterine artery

(Zemjanis, 1962).

Gestation diagnosis can also be performed by using transrectal ultrasound, which is a technique based on the use of ultrasound that allows the evaluation of genital structures (uterus and ovaries) (Racewicz et al., 2016). It evaluates the presence of the functional corpus luteum that appears in the ovary (Wang et al., 2020). It can be performed from day 26 after service.

In addition to being used for gestation diagnosis, they also use it for monitoring multiple gestations and evaluating fetal development (Ealy and Seekford, 2019). This technique allows the detection of twin gestations as early as 30 days post-insemination. In non-pregnant females, it can be used to identify the stage of the estrous cycle of the cow or to diagnose uterine and ovarian pathology (Sice et al., 2022).

It is a technique with a sensitivity of 97% at 30 days post artificial insemination (Fricke et al., 2016a). It is currently considered the most viable method for the diagnosis of pregnancies because the results are immediate (Sice et al., 2022), being able to diagnose the presence or absence of signs of pregnancy, embryo viability and detection of embryonic losses (Racewicz et al., 2016).

Table 6. Gestational structures detected by ultrasound.

STRUCTURES	DAY INTERVAL	AVERAGE IN DAYS
Embryo	19-24	20
Heartbeat	19-24	21
Allantoic membrane	22-25	23
Curved appearance of the embryo	22-30	25
Spine	26-33	29
Outline of former members	28-31	29
Amnios	28-33	29
Ocular orbits	29-33	30
Outline of hind limbs	30-33	31
L appearance of the embryo	29-39	33
Placentomas	33-38	35
Hooves	42-49	45
Fetal movement	42-50	45
ribs	51-55	53

Retrieved from Sice et al. (2022).

III. HYPOTHESIS

Charolais cows induced with an estrus synchronization protocol and Fixed-Time Artificial Insemination obtain the same conception rate during the spring and fall seasons under tropical conditions.

IV. OBJECTIVES

4.1. General

- The objective was to evaluate the effect of the spring and fall seasons on the conception rate of Charolais cows subjected to an estrus synchronization protocol and fixed-time artificial insemination under tropical conditions.

4.2. Specific

- Collect ambient temperature and relative humidity data from the herd location.
- Construct the temperature-humidity index to determine the degree of heat stress in the animals.
- Determine conception rate and estrus expression rate.

V. MATERIALS AND METHODS

Animals and treatments

All procedures used were approved by the Bioethics and Animal Welfare Commission of the Faculty of Veterinary Medicine and Animal Husbandry of the University of Colima (Evaluation Record: No. 2/2022). The study was carried out with 48 Charolais cows located at 19°18'06 "N and 104°15'15 "W in a commercial ranch dedicated to beef production in the Municipality of Manzanillo, Colima (**Figure 1**), at an altitude of 382 m asl, with a tropical climate (Köppen Cfb; García, 2004).

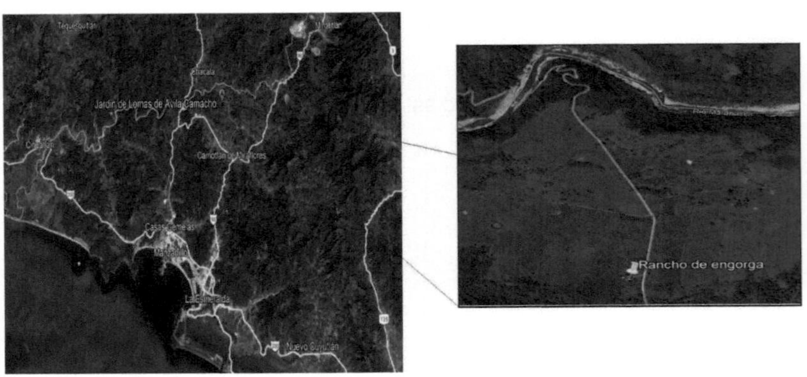

Figure 10. Location of commercial beef production ranch.

The study had a duration of 140 days divided into two periods of 70 d/epoch. The first period was during the fall season (November 14, 2021 to January 09, 2022) and the second period was during the spring season (April 10, 2022 to June 18, 2022). To start the study, body condition of 7 (where 1 is extremely wasted and 9 is extremely obese, (NASEM, 2016) days in milk (80 ± 20 d) and number of calvings (3 ± 1 calvings) were considered as selection criteria. Cows were randomly assigned to one of two epochs: 1) 26, cows in the fall; 2) 22, cows in the spring. Ten days before starting the synchronization protocol (d -10), signs of health were observed during clinical examination of the reproductive system of the females using a real-time transrectal ultrasound (iScan, Draminski®, Olsztyn, Poland), equipped with 7.5-Mhz transducer. Indeed, the presence of follicles ≥ 2 mm confirmed ovarian activity (Lucy et al., 1992). Additionally, the size of the uterus was evaluated to observe its complete involution.

The cows were under the same feeding regimen based on llanero and Tanzania grass (*Andropogon gayanus* and *Panicum maximum,* respectively) in an extensive system, common salt was provided as a mineral supplement and water *ad libitum.* The management pen was 15 m wide and 30 m long, with 3 m high shade in the center, covering only a small portion of the pen.

Estrus synchronization protocol

All cows were synchronized based on P_4 , which was released through a bovine intravaginal device (DIBActive 600® ; 0.6 g P_4 **DIB**), then 2 mg/mL IM estradiol benzoate (EstroActive® ; 1 mg/mL **BE**) was administered on day 0. On day 7 the DIB was removed and 0.150 mg cloprostenol (InducelActive® ; 0.075 mg/mL **CLO**), 0.5 mg estradiol cypionate (CipioActive® ; 1 mg/mL **ECP**), as well as 400 IU equine chorionic gonadotropin (GonActive; 200 IU/mL **eCG**) were administered intramuscularly. All hormonal products used in this estrus synchronization protocol were from the same commercial laboratory (Virbac, Zapopan, Jalisco, Mexico). Finally, fixed-time artificial insemination (**FTAI**) occurred 48 h later (**Figure 2**).

Pregnancy diagnosis

Pregnancy diagnosis was performed 39 d after IATF via transrectal ultrasound for each cow in both experiments. Additionally, conception rate (**CT**) was determined from the heartbeat of an embryo, as well as the presence of embryogenic fluid. Finally, prior to IATF, cervical mucus was observed in all cows to determine the rate of estrous expression.

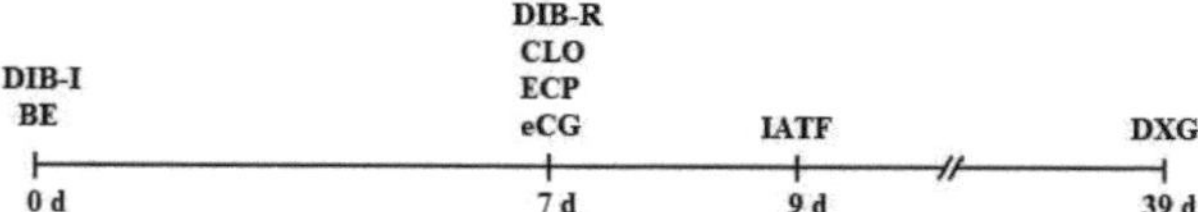

Figure 11. Estrus synchronization protocol. DIB-I and DIB-R = bovine intravaginal device insertion (I) and removal (R); BE = 2 mg estradiol benzoate; CLO = 0.150 mg cloprostenol; ECP = 0.5 mg estradiol cypionate; eCG = 400 IU equine chorionic gonadotropin; IATF = fixed-time artificial insemination; DXG = diagnosis of gestation.

Climatic variables

The climatic variables ambient temperature (**TA**, °C) and relative humidity (**RH**, %) were recorded every fifteen minutes during the study time. The data were obtained from the meteorological station of the National Laboratory of Modeling and Remote Sensing of the National Institute of Forestry, Agriculture and Livestock Researchers (INIFAP), located in the town of Manuel Avila Camacho in Manzanillo, Colima. With the variables obtained, the temperature-humidity index (**TIH**) was calculated as an indicator of EC with the following formula (Hahn, 1999):

$$ITTH = 0.81\ TTA + HR\ (\alpha\alpha\ - 14.4) + 46.4$$

Where:

$ITTH$ = temperature-humidity index;

TA = daily ambient temperature (°C); and

HR = daily relative humidity (%).

Statistical analysis

All statistical analyses were performed using SAS (2004) statistical software procedures. Maximum and minimum values corresponding to climatic variables such as, TA, HR and ITH were obtained using the Var procedure. The conception rate and estrus expression rate were analyzed by a Chi test of independence[2] using the Freq procedure. The statistical significance level was declared at 5% and trend between 5 and 10%.

VI. RESULTS

Figure 12 shows the maximum and minimum values of the ITH, RH and TA recorded during five weeks in the first period of the study, corresponding to the autumn season.

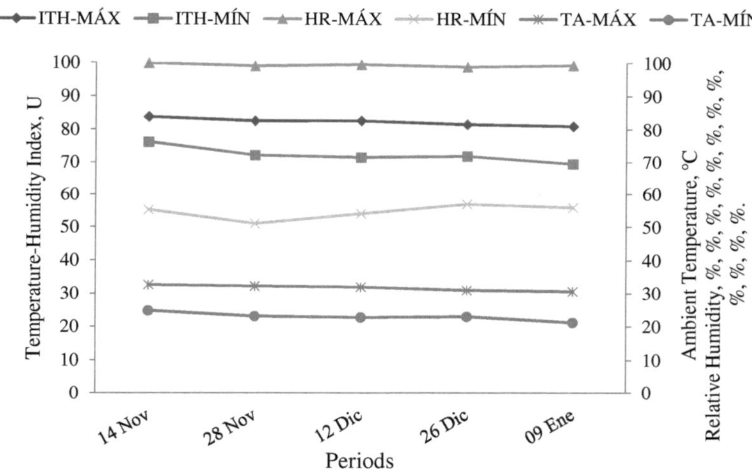

Maximum and minimum values of the temperature-humidity index, ambient temperature and relative humidity during the study period in autumn.

The highest value of the maximum average HTI was 83.8 units and the lowest was 81.0 units, during the first period of the study and the minimum value in the fifth period. In the same way, the minimum ITH was the highest value during the first period at 76.2 units, while in the fifth period it was 69.5 units as the lowest value.

For maximum RH values, the high value was 99.8% in the first period and the low value was 98.8% in the fourth period. Likewise, the minimum high and low RH values were 56.8 and 51.0 % during the fourth and second periods, respectively.

Finally, the maximum high and low TA values were 32.7 and 30.6 °C, in the first and last periods. On the other hand, the minimum high and low TA values were 24.8 and 21.3 °C in the same periods reported in maximum TA, respectively.

The ITH, RH and TA data were expressed in **Figure 13**. These results were recorded equally in five periods, corresponding to spring weather.

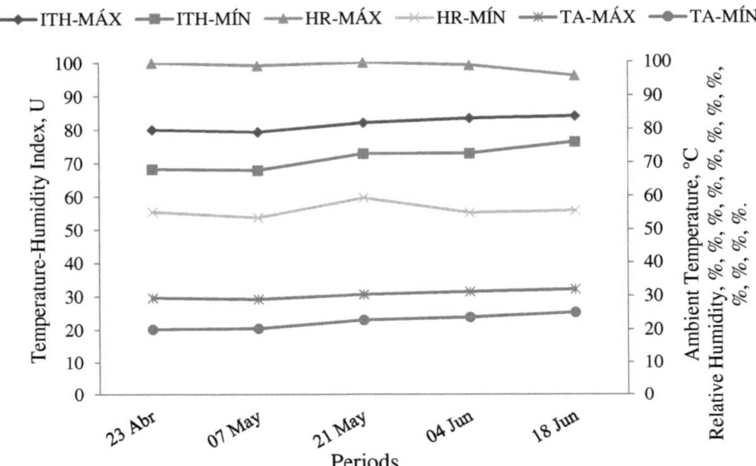

Maximum and minimum values of the temperature-humidity index, ambient temperature and relative humidity during the study period in spring.

The highest value of the maximum HTI was 83.9 units and the lowest was 79.3 units, during the fifth period of study and the minimum value in the second period. In the same way, the highest value of the minimum HTI was 76.1 units during the fifth period, while the lowest value was 67.9 units during the second period.

For maximum RH values, the high values were 100 % in the first and third periods, while the low value was 95.9 % in the fifth period. Likewise, the minimum high and low RH values were 59.5 and 53.7 % during the third and second periods, respectively.

Finally, the maximum high and low TA values were 32.0 and 29.2 °C, in the last and second periods. On the other hand, the minimum high and low TA values were 25.1 and 20.2 °C in the last and first period, respectively. It is worth mentioning that during the second period the TA was practically the same as the previous one with 20.5 °C.

Other maximum and minimum ITH, RH and TA values were recorded hourly during the study time. Fall values are shown in **Figure 14**, while spring values are shown in **Figure 15**.

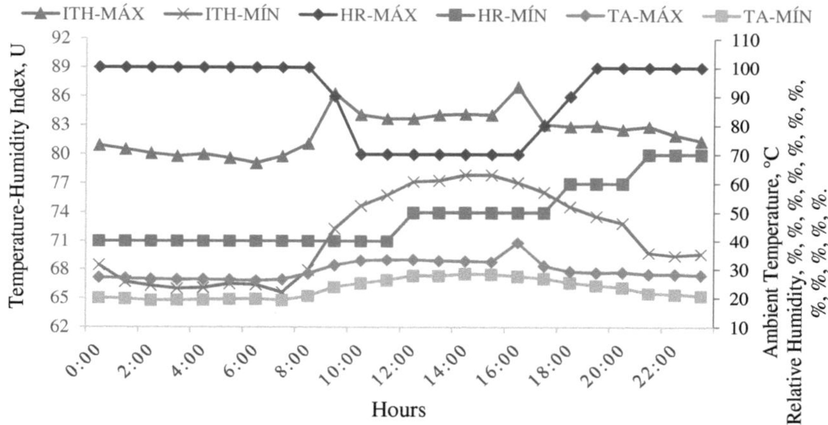

Maximum and minimum values of the temperature-humidity index (TIH), ambient temperature (TA) and relative humidity (RH) per hour during the study period in autumn.

The maximum ITH values recorded from 09:00 to 16:00 h, reached an average of 85 units. From 17:00 to 00:00 h, it reached an average of 82 units. From 01:00 to 08:00 h, an average of 80 units was recorded. The minimum ITH values recorded in the same time periods indicated above averaged 76, 72 and 67 units, respectively.

The maximum RH values recorded from 09:00 to 16:00 h, reached an average of 72.5 %. From 17:00 to 00:00 h, it reached an average of 96.2 %. From 01:00 to 08:00 h, an average of 100 % was recorded. The minimum RH values recorded in the same time periods indicated above averaged 46, 60 and 40 %, respectively.

The maximum TA values recorded from 09:00 to 16:00 h, reached an average of 34 °C. From 17:00 to 00:00 h, it reached an average of 29 °C. From 01:00 to 08:00 h, an average of 26 °C was recorded. The minimum TA values recorded in the same time periods indicated above averaged 27, 23 and 19 °C, respectively.

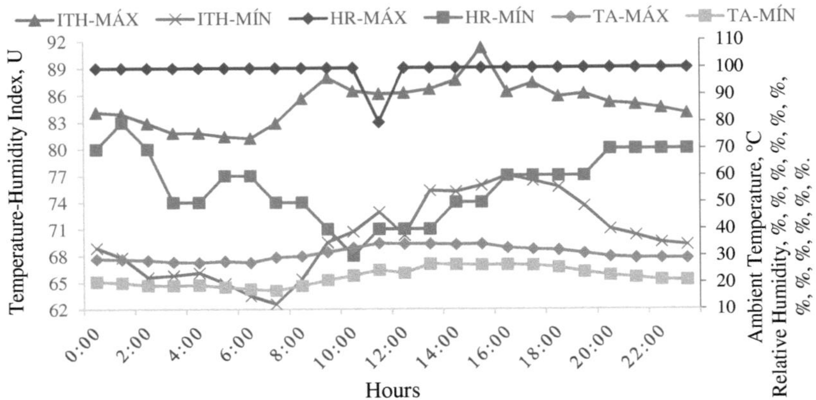

Maximum and minimum values of the temperature-humidity index (TIH), ambient temperature (TA) and relative humidity (RH) per hour during the study period in spring.

The maximum ITH values recorded from 09:00 to 16:00 h, reached an average of 87 units. From 17:00 to 00:00 h, it reached an average of 85 units. From 01:00 to 08:00 h, an average of 83 units was recorded. The minimum ITH values recorded in the same time periods indicated above averaged 74, 72 and 66 units, respectively.

The maximum RH values recorded from 12:00 to 10:00 h, reached an average of 100 %. Only during 11:00 h it reached 80 %. The minimum RH values recorded from 09:00 to 16:00 h, reached an average of 44 %. From 17:00 to 00:00 h, it reached an average of 66 %. From 01:00 to 08:00 h, an average of 59 % was recorded.

The maximum TA values recorded from 09:00 to 16:00 h, reached an average of 34 °C. From 17:00 to 00:00 h, it reached an average of 30 °C. From 01:00 to 08:00 h, an average of 28 °C was recorded. The minimum TA values recorded in the same time periods indicated above averaged 25, 23 and 19 °C, respectively.

Table 7 shows the results obtained in conception rate and estrus expression rate in spring compared to fall. The conception rate tended to be higher ($P<0.10$) during the fall, since 61.5 % was obtained, while during the spring it was 36.4 %. Also the estrus expression rate tended to be higher ($P<0.10$) during autumn with 54.4 % compared to spring, obtaining 31.8 %.

Table 7. Effect of season on conception rate and estrus expression of Charolais cows under fixed-time artificial insemination in the tropics.

Epoch	TC[1]	TEE[2]
Spring	36.4 (8/22)[a]	31.8 (7/22)[a]
Autumn	61.5 (16/26)[b]	54.5 (12/22)[b]

[ab]Different literals indicate statistical trend ($P<0.10$).

[1]Conception rate, %;[2] Estrus expression rate, %.

VII. DISCUSSION

CE is generated when changes occur in the environment that exceed the thermoneutral or animal welfare zone (Armstrong, 1994). The best TA conditions in cattle are 18 ºC (Pires, 2003). Chemineau (1993) commented that cattle after being subjected to high temperatures use evaporative methods such as respiratory rate and sweating, which generate a high energy expenditure to try to lose heat.

AT is associated with RH (Jeelani et al., 2018). In fact, it is considered that, if TA and RH exceed 25 °C and 60%, respectively; animals could reach up to 73 ITH units to get out of the comfort zone and present problems to maintain homeostasis.

The averages obtained in maximum TA during the autumn study period showed practically no variation between each period. During the first three time periods it remained at 32 °C, approximately; while in the last two periods it remained an average of 31 °C. During the spring, the first two periods recorded 29 °C; from the third, fourth and fifth periods on, it increased by 1 °C, each time. In general, the climate in the municipality of Manzanillo, Col. is tropical, however, during the autumn months, the climate becomes dry and slightly less hot, with temperatures that oscillate between 29 °C. During the summer months, the climate is rainy with TA ranging from 32 °C; the month with the lowest ambient temperatures is March, ranging from 19 to 23 °C (METEORED, 2022).

Zazueta et al. (2021) in their study conducted in Sinaloa, Mexico, show that in the fall season the maximum TA obtained were 32.8 ºC and the minimum 18.2ºC. The maximum temperatures coincide with the current study; however, the minimum temperatures are 5 °C lower, i.e., in the study an average of 23 °C was reached. Therefore, in spite of presenting that temperatures could be more favorable for cattle during the fall, the reality is that environmental conditions are hostile in the region of Manzanillo, Colima.

Cattle have the ability to thermoregulate and regulate body temperature. Habeeb et al. (2018) mention that animals that have been exposed to intense heat conditions show an increase in cortisol concentration, which is directly related to the presence of heat stress. During the time of the study, it was possible to observe that the AT in both periods of the study presented an average of 30 ºC. However, when obtaining the results by hour, it was observed that during autumn the average maximum RT was above 31 ºC, for at least 9 h.

During the spring 11 h (0900-1900 h) recorded average maximum TA above 31 °C, however, from 1100-1500 h they exceeded 34.0 °C. During the afternoon the TA recorded high values; the morning and evening values in both seasons ranged from 26 to 29 °C. Therefore, the cattle used in the present study were particularly stressed during the most hostile hours of the day, however, in reality, the hours of sun exposure exceeded 12 h.

In the case of beef cattle, high temperatures increase water consumption, decrease feed intake and affect meat yield (Arias et al., 2008). High temperatures alter cattle metabolism and generate a hormonal imbalance that prevents adequate reproduction (Bañuelos and Sánchez, 2005). On the other hand, the age at puberty can be affected by low EC, since feed intake and grazing hours decrease, which causes the animal not to obtain the nutritional requirements during growth and delays the time to puberty. Therefore, increasing uterine temperature by 0.5 °C, above 38.6 °C (normal), results in a 12.8% reduction in pregnancy rate (Gwazdauskas et al., 1973).

If the AT drops at night below 21 °C for 3 to 6 h, cows lose at night all the heat gained during the day (Correa et al., 2016). In fact, this did not happen during the fall, because, in the night hours, ambient temperatures remained within 28 °C (1000 - 0000 h), then decreased to 26 °C (0100 to 700 h). Therefore, it is important to consider that the ITH never dropped below 79 units throughout the fall, which indicates light EC in cattle, since they were not able to mitigate the heat they received during the course of the day.

During the spring, the ITH never dropped below 83 units, therefore, a moderate EC was obtained in the animals. Ambient temperatures were higher than 30 °C. The relevance of this scenario is that the cows during this period were exposed to this temperature for at least 11 h, and it negatively affected the heat mitigation and thermoregulation of the cattle.

Thompson et al. (1996) reported that the decrease in conception rate in the hot season varies 20-30% less than in the rainy or winter season. Now, when considering the above in this study, during the spring a 69% decrease was obtained with respect to the fall, that is, 30% higher than that reported in the literature. Therefore, it is evident that the heat load expressed in the conception rate obtained by spring cows was higher. High TA can cause the death of cows under CE (Rhoads et al., 2013). One of the strategies that help mitigate high TA is to place shaded areas, which can be adequate depending on the number of animals and their location; in fact, it has been shown that animals decrease heat load under shade by 30 to 45% compared to animals that were directly exposed to solar radiation (Ulvshammar, 2014).

The ITH has been used to indicate the degree of CD in cattle, in which the values of HR and TA are combined (Romo et al., 2019). In the current study, the maximum values of ITH during both epochs, did not decrease from 80 units on average. The highest values of ITH in both epochs were those registered during 0900 to 1600 h. In fact, during spring it reached 87 units on average, however, during autumn 2 units less were obtained. Nevertheless, during the 1600 h of autumn an average maximum ITH of 87 units was obtained, leaving the cows in a moderate EC, while during the 1500 h of spring an average maximum ITH of 92 units was obtained, which is 5 units of deference made the cows experience severe EC. During the spring it was feasible to obtain an 8 % difference between the total average maximum ITH value recorded per hour, which was 85 units, and the average maximum ITH value recorded at 1500 h which was 92 units. Huertas et al. (2020), comments that, if the ITH values are between 82 and greater than 92 units, moderate to severe CD may occur, which could influence the reproductive efficiency of cattle. An improvement in comfort allows animals to allocate more time in grazing and ruminating activities to obtain a better conception rate (Peri et al., 2016). An example of this is when animals of both epochs could have found during the night hours a relief to consume feed and mitigate energy demands intended for maintenance and reproduction, however, this was not evaluated during the study.

On the other hand, in **Figure 12** it was possible to observe an elevation of 11 units of maximum ITH above 72 units (value without EC; Macías et al., 2018) at least during the first three study periods in autumn. Now, the same happened in spring season, i.e., 11 units of ITH above the value without EC were also obtained, but during the last two study periods in spring.

Hahn et al. (1999) mention that it is not only important to take into account the ITH score, but also the duration and intensity of the ITH (number of hours/days/frequency of exposure, etc.). The frequency of exposure is of great importance because the more hours of exposure, the less time the animals have to dissipate the heat load (St-Pierre et al., 2013).

The minimum values of ITH in the fall and spring season (**Figure 12** and **13**), hover between 67.9 and 69.5 units, that is, a difference of about 1 °C, which in this case does not generate light CE, however, these values were recorded between the morning hours (0600 and 0700 h; **Figure 14** and **15**). This could generate controversy, because there are only two hours of the day in which the cattle in the study were found without the presence of some type of heat stress, however, it is known that two hours does not generate sufficient relief. Huertas et al. 2020, mention that heat stress levels in cattle are considered normal if the ITH is less than 72 units, i.e. between 72 to 78 units is a mild CE, between 79 to 83 units is a moderate CE and greater than 84 units is severe. Additionally, Correa et al., (2016) mention that if the ITH units are above 72 units the conception rate is reduced up to 50%, due to CE. This coincides with the moderate CE values during the fall, as there was a 39% reduction in conception rate in the study cows; however, during the spring this reduction was higher at 64 %, as a result of severe CE. This means that, if ITH values are elevated, it can also increase physiological constants in cattle (Mader et al., 2006), such as respiratory rate, heart rate, decreased feed intake, increased water consumption and imbalances in blood gas and plasma electrolytes (Carroll and Forsberg, 2007).

In cows with CD, the duration of estrus is reduced and the incidence of anestrus increases (Collier et al., 2017). Heat stress affects estrus duration and intensity, hormonally, blood flow, and embryo development. Naturally, physical inactivity or prostration serves to decrease the heat load on the animal, however, it is the main cause of a low estrus detection rate, as it hinders the work of estrus observers (Góngora and Hernández, 2010). As body temperature increases, the embryo loses its vitality and resorption is generated (Fournel et al., 2017). Therefore, it is logical to think that all those animals that have greater comfort and productivity are those in cooler environments with respect to those in warm places (Damian and Fernandez, 2021). According to the results of this study it is possible to implement strategies that help mitigate the effects of EC, especially in the spring, probably using silvopastoral systems, where Mancera et al. (2018), comment that in addition to providing food for the animals, they provide a natural protection against solar radiation because this helps in an integral way to balance the natural and forage components, allowing to diversify the ecosystem (Viñoles et al., 2022). Additionally, reproductive management strategies can be carried out at times with lower heat load, making modifications in the corrals that include more shaded areas or even making environmental modifications based on cooling systems, since by using them, it has been possible to reduce the ITH from 1 to 6 units, the TA from 0.2 to 5 °C (Fournel et al., 2017), and even improve the fertility rate by 40% (Correa et al., 2016).

Factors affecting the rate of estrous expression include environmental, health, nutritional and social problems (Butler and Smith, 1989). Therefore, the negative effects of CE in cattle are associated with reduced estrus intensity (Younas et al., 1993), decreased estrous expression in cattle presents changes in ovarian function. This was evidenced in the study, since this variable tended to be greater in autumn than in spring, i.e., during spring it was reduced by 68%, but during autumn only 46%, which evidences the comfort or hostility of each season, respectively.

The use of estrus synchronization and IATF are alternatives that help improve the reproduction of cattle under CE, since it eliminates the need to detect estrus to increase the pregnancy rate and reproductive efficiency (Nezhad, 2013). Then, increasing the rate of estrus detection could improve reproductive parameters in production units (Saumande and Humblot, 2005). The use of IATF does not protect the embryo from embryonic mortality caused by CD (De la Sota et al., 1998). Espinoza et al. (2021), conducted a study with 110 cows to evaluate estrous response and gestation in *Bos taurus* beef cows, where two treatments were used, the first treatment for ovulation of the cows was based on estradiol benzoate (IM, 2 mg) and at the same time the insertion of a vaginal device (IVD) with 1.3 g of P_4 , this at day 0. The IVD was removed after 8 days and 25 mg of PGF2α, 1 mg of estradiol cypionate (EC) and 300 IU of equine chorionic gonadotropin (eCG) were applied, at 48 to 52 hours later the IATF was performed. The second treatment was similar to treatment 1, but without including eCG.

Results of 73 % in gestation rate and 75 % response in estrous expression rate were obtained in cows that received eCG treatment, however, in cows that did not use eCG, the estrous expression rate was 57 % and the gestation rate was 53 %, which considerably decreased the percentage of cows that were not induced with eGC. The results obtained in the study of Espinoza et al. (2021), are above those obtained during the fall and spring time, i.e. 38 and 136 %, respectively, despite the fact that in the current study the IATF protocol counted with the administration of eCG.

Some producers consider that the additional management derived from the application of IATF protocols may increase the level of CD in animals, however, in this study no increase was shown as a consequence of management during the implementation of IATF.

Environmental modifications based on cooling systems can help mitigate the negative effects of heat stress in beef cattle.

VIII. CONCLUSION

Conception rate and estrous expression tended to improve during the fall relative to the spring. Heat stress conditions were moderate during the fall, but severe in the spring. Both times can seriously compromise reproductive parameters of Charolais cows under fixed-time artificial insemination in the tropics.

IX. LITERATURE CITED

1. Anta E, *et al.* (1989). Analysis of published information on bovine reproduction in Mexico. *Veterinaria Mexico*, 20, 11-18. ISSN 2448-6760.
2. Alvarez, V., *et al.* (2020). Effect of prepartum supplementation with calcium chloride on glucose and urea concentration in the calving-estrus interval in Carora cows. *Veterinary Science Gazette*, *25*(2), 15-25. Available: https://revistas.uclave.org/index.php/gcv/article/view/3731
3. Arias, R,. *et al.* (2008). Climatic factors affecting productive performance of beef and dairy cattle. *Archives of Veterinary Medicine*, 40(1), 7-22. http://dx.doi.org/10.4067/S0301-732X2008000100002
4. Armstrong, D. (1994). Heat stress interaction with shade and cooling. *Journal of Dairy Science*, 77, 2044-2050. https://doi.org/10.3168/jds.S0022-0302(94)77149-6.
5. Aro, R. A., & Álvarez, R. J. A. (2019). Effect of GnRH in stages of estrus synchronization protocol with progestogens and fixed-time artificial insemination in crossbred Zebu cows. *Apthapi*, 5(1), 1380-1389. Available: https://apthapi.umsa.bo/index.php/ATP/article/view/15
6. Avalos, D.O.Y., *et al.* (2018). Fixed-time artificial insemination in cows with prolonged proestrus of 60 and 72 hours. Agronomia Mesoamericana, 29(2), 363-373. http://dx.doi.org/10.15517/ma.v29i2.29503
7. Bañuelos, R., & Sánchez, S. (2005). The heat stress protein HSP70 functions as an indicator of bovine adaptation to arid zones. *REDVET*, 6 (3),12. Available: http://www.veterinaria.org/revistas/redvet/n030305.html
8. Bartolomé, J. (2009). Endocrinology and physiology of gestation and parturition in cattle. *Taurus*, 11, 20-28. Available: http://www.produccion-animal.com.ar/
9. Becker, C., et al. (2020). Invited review: Physiological and behavioral effects of heat stress in dairy cows. *Journal of Dairy Science*, 103(8), 6751-70. https://doi.org/10.3168/jds.2019-17929
10. Boeta, M., *et al.* (2018). Artificial insemination. Valencia, J. Reproductive physiology of domestic animals (1st Edition, pp. 265-283). *Mexico: FMVZ-UNAM.* ISBN: 9786073006712

11. Brito, R. (1999). Fisiologia de la Reproduccion Animal con elementos de Biotecnologia" *Editorial Felix Varela*, Havana. pp. 254- 261.
12. Butler, W., & Smith, R. (1989). Interrelationships between energy balance and post partum reproductive function. *Journal of Dairy Science,* 72, 767-87. https://doi.org/10.3168/jds.S0022-0302(89)79169-4
13. Carroll, J., & Forsberg, N. (2007). Influence of stress and nutrition on cattle immunity. *Veterinary Clinics of North America: Food Animal Practice*, 23(1), 105-149. https://doi.org/10.1016/j.cvfa.2007.01.003
14. Carvalho, B., *et al.* (2008). Effect of early luteolysis in progesterone-based timed AI protocols in *Bos indicus, Bos indicus* x *Bos taurus*, and *Bos taurus* heifers. *Theriogenology*, 69(2), 167-175. https://doi.org/10.1016/j.theriogenology.2007.08.035
15. Cattle, E. (2020). Reproductive parameters and reproductive efficiency in beef cattle. Available: http://repository.ucc.edu.co/bitstream/20.500.12494/17465/1/2020_parametros_reproductivos_eficiencia.pdf
16. Chemineau, P. (1993). Environment and animal reproduction. Available: http://www.fao.org/3/v1650t04.html
17. Colazo, M., & Mapletoft, J. (2022). Factors associated with gonadotropin release and ovulation following exogenous GnRH administration in *Bos taurus. Veterinary Science*, *24*(2), 221-240. https://cerac.unlpam.edu.ar/index.php/veterinaria/article/view/7000/7637
18. Collier, R., *et al.* (2017). 100-Year Review: stress physiology including heat stress. *Journal of Dairy Science*, 100, 1036780. https://doi.org/10.3168/jds.2017-13676
19. Correa, A., *et al.* (2016). Effect of time of progesterone supplementation on serum progesterone and the conception rate of cooled Holstein heifers during the summer. *Animal Science Journal*, 87(6), 745-749. https://doi.org/10.1111/asj.12488
20. Damián, M., & Fernández, D. (2021). Thermoregulatory effect of Merino Isla Socorro sheep and their crosses with Pelibuey at two times of the year under tropical conditions. *Faculty of Veterinary Medicine and Animal Husbandry, University of Colima.*

21. Davidson, A. P., & Stabenfeldt, G. H. (2014). Section VI: Reproduction and lactation. Control of ovulation and the corpus luteum. Reproductive cycles. In J. G. Cunningham & B. G. Klein (Eds.), *Cunningham's Textbook of Veterinary Physiology* (4th illus., Vol. 1, pp. 416-430). *Barcelona, Spain: Elsevier Health Science Division.* ISBN 9781437723618.
22. de Aguiar, D., *et al.* (2020). Heat stress impairs in vitro development of preantral follicles of cattle. *Animal Reproduction Science*, 213, 106277. https://doi.org/10.1016/j.anireprosci.2020.106277. https://doi.org/10.1016/j.anireprosci.2020.106277
23. De la Sota, R. L., *et al.* (1998). Evaluation of timed insemination during summer heat stress in lactating dairy cattle. *Theriogenology*, 49(4), 761-770. https://doi.org/10.1016/S0093-691X(98)00025-9
24. Ealy, A. & Seekford, Z. (2019). Symposium review: predicting pregnancy loss in dairy cattle. *Journal of Dairy Science*, 102(12), 11798-11804. https://doi.org/10.3168/jds.2019-17176
25. Espinoza, V.J.L., *et al.* (2021). Fixed-time artificial insemination and reinsemination of beef cows treated with and without equine chorionic gonadotropin. *Nova Scientia*, 13(27). https://doi.org/10.21640/ns.v13i27.2747
26. FAO. (2017). Food and agriculture organization of the united nations. Available: http://www.fao.org/mexico/fao-en-mexico/mexico-en-una-mirada/en/ (December 2017).
27. Fernández, S. M. C. (2008). Ovogenesis, folliculogenesis and follicular dynamics. In S. M. C. Fernández (Ed.), El ciclo estral de la vaca: diagnóstico fotográfico (1st illustrated ed., Vol. 1, pp. 10-18). Zaragoza, Spain: *Servet Diseño y Comunicación.* ISBN: 978-84-935971-2-2.
28. FIRA. (2017). Panorama agroalimentario. Beef and veal 2017. From trusts instituted in relation to agriculture. Available: https://www.gob.mx/cms/uploads/attachment/file/200639/Panorama_Agroalimentario_Carne_de_bovino_2017__1_.pdf (December 6, 2017). [Links]
29. Fournel, S., *et al.* (2017). Practices for alleviating heat stress of dairy cows in humid continental climates: a literature review. *Animals*, 7(5), 37. https://doi.org/10.3390/ani7050037

30. Fricke, M., *et al.* (2016a). Effect of manipulating progesterone before timed artificial insemination 50 on reproductive and endocrine parameters in seasonal-calving, pasturebased Holstein-Friesian cows. *Journal of Dairy* Science, 99(8), 6780-92. https://doi.org/10.3168/jds.2016-11229
31. Fricke, P., et al. (2016b). Methods for and Imple-mentation of Pregnancy Diagnosis in Dairy Cows. *Veterinary Clinics: Food Animal Practice*, 32(1), 165-180. https://doi.org/10.1016/j.cvfa.2015.09.006.
32. Gallegos, F., *et al.* (2022). Bovine in vitro Embryo Production: State of the Art Bovine Embryo Production in vitro: State of the Art. *ESPOCH Congresses: The Ecuadorian Journal of STEAM*, *2*(1). http://dx.doi.org/10.18502/espoch.v2i2.11192
33. García, E. (2004). Modifications to the Köppen climate classification system. *National Autonomous University of Mexico*. ISBN 9683673988
34. Giraldo, J. (2014). A look at the use of artificial insemination in cattle. *Revista Lasallista de Investigación*, 4 (1) pp.51-57. Available: http://www.redalyc.org/articulo.oa?id=69540108
35. Giraldo, J., *et al.* (2017). Evaluation of ovarian stimulation and quality of bovine oocytes obtained by follicular aspiration. *Journal of Agriculture and Animal Sciences*, 6(1), 20- 28. http://dx.doi.org/10.22507/jals.v6n1a2
36. Gómez, T., *et al.* (2014). The two hypothalamic orexin peptides: Their location and action on the hypothalamic-pituitary-gonadal axis. *Mexican Journal of Neuroscience*, 15(6), 345-350. Available: https://www.medigraphic.com/pdfs/revmexneu/rmn-2014/rmn146g.pdf
37. Góngora, A., & Hernández, A. (2010). Cow reproduction is affected by high environmental temperatures. *Revista UDCA Actualidad & Divulgación Científica*, 13(2), 163-173. https://doi.org/10.31910/rudca.v13.n2.2010.742
38. Granados, D., *et al.* (2018). Characterization and typification of the dual purpose system in cattle ranching in rural development district 151, tabasco, Mexico. *Acta Universitaria*, *28*(6), 47-57. https://doi.org/10.15174/au.2018.1916
39. Gutiérrez, J., *et al.* (2005). Use of the ovsynch protocol in the control of postpartum anestrus in dual-purpose crossbred cows. *Revista Científica*, 15(1), 7-13. Available: http://www.redalyc.org/articulo.oa?id=95915102

40. Gwazdauskas, F., *et al.* (1973). Physiological, environmental, and hormonal factors at insemination which may affect conception. *Journal of Dairy Science* 56 (7), 873-877. https://doi.org/10.3168/jds.S0022-0302(73)85270-1.
41. Habeeb, A., *et al.* (2018). Negative effects of heat stress on growth and milk production of farm animals. *Journal of Animal Husbandry and Dairy Science*, 2(1), 1-12. Available: https://www.sryahwapublications.com/journal-of-animal-husbandry-and-dairy-science/pdf/v2-i1/1.pdf
42. Hafez, E. S. E., & Hafez, B. (2002). Folliculogenesis, oocyte maturation and ovulation. Hafez, E. S. E., & Hafez, B. (Eds.). Artificial reproduction and insemination in animals (4th Edition, pp. 70-83). *McGraw-Hill Interamericana Editores, S. A. de C. V.* ISBN. 9701037197
43. Hahn, G. J. (1999). Dynamic responses of cattle to thermal heat loads. *Journal of Animal Science*, 77(suppl_2), 10-20. https://doi.org/10.2527/1997.77suppl_210x. https://doi.org/10.2527/1997.77suppl_210x
44. Hernández C., J. (2012). Clinical physiology of dairy cattle reproduction. *Mexico, UNAM.* https://doi.org/10.22201/fmvz.9786070286902e.2016
45. Horrach, M., *et al.* (2021). Factors affecting conception rate in fixed-time insemination in crossbred cows. *Journal of Animal Production*, *33*(1), 26-36. Available: https://revistas.reduc.edu.cu/index.php/rpa/article/view/e3576
46. Huertas, S., *et al.* (2020). Valuation of temperature and humidity index as a reliable measure to evaluate heat stress in cattle in temperate silvopastoral systems. *National Institute of Agricultural Research.* Available: http://www.ainfo.inia.uy/digital/bitstream/item/14475/1/Inia-Fpta-87-proyecto-311-2020.pdf#page=57
47. INEGI. (2020). National yearbook. Available: https://cuentame.inegi.org.mx/monografias/informacion/col/territorio/#:~:text=Por%20su%20superficie%2C%20Colima%20ocupa%20el%20lugar%2028%20a%20nivel%20nacional.&text=Colima%20tiene%20una%20extensi%C3%B3n%20de,de%20Poblaci%C3%B3n%20y%20Vivienda%202020

48. INTAGRI (2018). Reproductive characteristics of the bovine female. Available: https://www.intagri.com/articulos/ganaderia/caracteriticas-reproductivas-de-la-hembrabovina
49. Jiménez, J., & Sánchez, R. (2014). "The beef market in Mexico, 1970-2011." Social Studies. *Journal of Contemporary Food and Regional Development*, 22 (43). Available: https://www.scielo.org.mx/pdf/estsoc/v22n43/v22n43a4.pdf
50. Jeelani, R., *et al.* (2018). Reassessment of temperature-humidity index for measuring heat stress in crossbred dairy cattle of a sub-tropical region. *Journal of Thermal Biology*, 82, 99-106. https://doi.org/10.1016/j.jtherbio.2019.03.017.
51. Kruif, A. (1978). Factors influencing the fertility of a cattle population. *Reproduction*, 54, 507-518. https://doi.org/10.1530/jrf.0.0540507.
52. López, H. (2021). Early diagnosis and confirmation of gestation. *BM Editores, SA de CV.* Available: https://bmeditores.mx/ganaderia/diagnostico-temprano-y-confirmacion-de-la-gestacion/#:~:text=El%20diagn%C3%B3stico%20temprano%20de%20la,vaca%20est%C3%A1%20o%20no%20pre%C3%B1ada
53. Lozano, R., *et al.* (1992). Effect of environment on reproductive behavior and fertility of Swiss American breed cows in the subhumid tropics. *Revista Mexicana de Ciencias Pecuarias*, 30 (3), 208-222. Available: https://cienciaspecuarias.inifap.gob.mx/index.php/Pecuarias/article/view/3621
54. Loyo, A., *et al.* (2018) Evaluation of productive and reproductive parameters in *Bos taurus* x *Bos indicus* crossbred cattle in dual purpose system in Veracruz. *Innovación en la Ganadería Veracruzana*, 183. Available: http://cdigital.uv.mx/handle/123456789/39961
55. Lucy, M., *et al.* (1992). Factors that affect ovarian follicular dynamics in cattle. *Journal of Animal Science*, 70(11), 3615-3626. https://doi.org/10.2527/1992.70113615x.
56. Macias , U., et al. (2018). Variations in thermoregulatory responses of hair sheep during summer months in a desert climate. *Revista Mexicana de Ciencias Pecuarias*, 9(4), 739-753. https://doi.org/10.22319/rmcp.v9i4.4527
57. Mader, T., *et al.* (2006). Environmental Factors Influencing Heat Stress in Feedlot Cattle. *Journal of Animal Science*, 84, 712-719. https://doi.org/10.2527/2006.843712x

58. Mancera, K., *et al.* (2018). Integrating links between tree coverage and cattle welfare in silvopastoral systems evaluation. *Agronomy for Sustainable Development,* 38, 1-9. https://doi.org/10.1007/s13593-018-0497-3. https://doi.org/10.1007/s13593-018-0497-3
59. Mapletoft, R. (2006). Embryo transfer in cattle. *IVIS Reviews in Veterinary medicine, I.V.I.S* (Ed.) *International Veterinary information Service, Ithaca NY*; R0104. 1196.EN
60. Marcoppido, G., *et al.* (2018). Animal welfare: stress response in cattle used in research. *USAL Research Yearbook,* (4). Available: https://p3.usal.edu.ar/index.php/anuarioinvestigacion/article/view/4209/5239
61. Marizancén, M., & Artunduaga, L. (2017). Genetic improvement in cattle through artificial insemination and fixed-time artificial insemination. *Revista de Investigación Agraria y Ambienta,* 8(2), 247-249. https://doi.org/10.22490/21456453.2050
62. Matamoros, R., & Sanhueza, J. (2017). Basic principles of the endocrine system. *Fundamentals of reproductive physiology and endocrinology in domestic animals, Ed. University of Santo Tomas, Santiago de Chile* 11 pp. ISBN: 9789560104106.
63. Mbuthia, J., *et al.* (2021). Modeling heat stress effects on dairy cattle milk production in a tropical environment using test-day records and random regression models. *Animal,* 15(8), 100222. https://doi.org/10.1016/j.animal.2021.100222. https://doi.org/10.1016/j.animal.2021.100222
64. METEORED. Open Information System. Available: https://www.meteored.mx/clima_Manzanillo-America+Norte-Mexico-Colima-MMZO-1-22335.html.
65. Mikkola, M., & Taponen, J. (2017). Embryo yield in dairy cattle after superovulation with Folltropin or Pluset. Theriogenology, 88, 84-88. https://doi.org/10.1016/j.theriogenology.2016.09.052.
66. NASEM (2016). Nutrient requirements of beef cattle. National Academies of Sciences, Engineering, and Medicine. ISBN: 9780309317023
67. Navarro, M.M.C., *et al.* (2021a). Embryo transfer in domestic mammals. Rangel Santos, R. Reproducción asistida y conservación de mamíferos (1st Edition, pp. 64-81). *UAM-Ediciones del Lirio.* ISBN: 9786078785278

68. Navarro M. M. C., *et al.* (2021b). Assisted reproduction in mammalian conservation. Navarro M.M.C., *et al.* Assisted reproduction and mammal conservation (1st Edition, pp. 121-135). *UAM-Ediciones del Lirio.* ISBN. 9786078785278
69. Nezhad, F., *et al.* (2013). Effect of heat stress on oxidative reactions in the sheep sertoli cells. International *Journal of Agriculture and Crop Science*, 6.
70. Norman, J., *et al.* (2017). Selection of yield and fitness traits when culling Holsteins during the first three lactations. *Journal of Dairy Science*, 90, 1008-1020. https://doi.org/10.3168/jds.s0022-0302(07)71586-2.
71. Obando, S.D.A. (2020). Pharmacological basis and update on bovine estrus synchronization. Available: https://repository.ucc.edu.co/server/api/core/bitstreams/1da85936-9b0c-4c15-b8b2-bb1a679c0578/content
72. Food and Agriculture Organization of the United Nations (FAO) (1968), Physical Characteristics of the Charolais Breed, 2nd edition, *Wisconsin - United States*, pp. 353.
73. Palacios, N., *et al.* (2022). Distúrbios reprodutivos em bovinos leiteiros causados por estresse térmico Reproductive disorders in dairy cattle caused by heat stress. *Brazilian Journal of Animal and Environmental Research*, *5*(1), 1336-1341. https://doi.org/10.34188/bjaerv5n1-103.
74. Parra, I., & Magaña, Á. (2019). Techno-economic characteristics of bovine production systems based on introduced criollo breeds in Mexico. *Ecosistemas y Recursos Agropecuarios*, *6*(18), 535-547. https://doi.org/10.19136/era.a6n18.2160
75. Parra, M., et al. (2017). Superovulation with follicular wave synchronization and natural estrus in Holstein cows. *Journal of Animal Production*, 29(1), 41-44. Available: http://scielo.sld.cu/scielo.php?script=sci_arttext&pid=S2224-79202017000100008
76. Pérez, E., *et al.* (2022). Ovarian function and response to estrus synchronization in Criollo cattle in Mexico. Review. *Revista Mexicana de Ciencias Pecuarias*, *13*(2), 422-451. https://doi.org/10.22319/rmcp.v13i2.6032

77. Pérez, L., *et al.* (2015). Evaluation of two fixed-term artificial insemination protocols (FTAI) with two ovulation inducers (estradiol benzoate and estradiol cypionate) in Caqueteño Creole cows in the department of Caquetá. REDVET. *Electronic Journal of Veterinary Medicine*, 16(9), 1-11. Available: http://www.redalyc.org/articulo.oa?id=63641785003
78. Peri, P., *et al.* (2016). Silvopastoral Systems in the subtropical and temperature zones of South America: An Overview. In: Peri P, Dube F, Varella A. *Silvopastoral Systems in Southern South America,*1-8. https://doi.org/10.1007/978-3-319-24109-8_1
79. Pires, V., *et al.* (2021). Expression of candidate genes for residual feed intake in tropically adapted *Bos taurus* and *Bos indicus* bulls under thermoneutral and heat stress environmental conditions. *Journal of Thermal Biology*, 99, 102998. https://doi.org/10.1016/j.jtherbio.2021.102998
80. Pires, M. (2003). Relação dos dados climáticos com o desempenho animal. *Dados climáticos e sua utilização na atividade leiteira*, 1: 250. Available: https://www.embrapa.br/documents/1354377/1743402/Dados+Climaticos+-+Desempenho+Animal.pdf/2e7f5b68-39af-4405-8119-cd6f4a549746?version=1.0
81. Pohler, K., *et al.* (2017). Pregnancy Diagnosis in Cattle: when,why and how. *Proceedings, Applied Reproductive Strategies in Beef Cattle*, 181-192.
82. Puebla, S., *et al.* (2018). Determinants of regional beef supply in Mexico, 1994-2013. *Region and Society*, *30*(72). https://doi.org/10.22198/rys.2018.72.a895
83. Racewicz, P., *et al.* (2016). Ultrasonographic diagnosis of early pregnancy in cattle us-ing different ultrasound systems. *Tierärztliche Praxis Ausgabe G: Großtiere/Nutztiere*, 44(03), 151-156.
84. Ramirez, L. & Lílido, N. (2006). The hypothalamus of domestic mammals. *Livestock World,* 2(1), 16-17. Available: http://www.saber.ula.ve/bitstream/handle/123456789/21953/articulo_6.pdf?sequence=2&isAllowed=y#:~:text=El%20hipot%C3%A1lamo%20es%20asiento%20de,ante%20est%C3%ADmulos%20provenientes%20del%20ambiente.

85. Reece, W. O. (2015). Section IX: Endocrinology, reproduction, and lactation. Female Reproduction in Mammals. In W. O. Reece, H. H. Erickson, J. P. Goff, & E. E. E. Uemura (Eds.), Dukes' *Physiology of Domestic Animals* (13th illustrated ed., Vol. 1, pp. 670-693). New York, United States: WileyBlackwell. ISBN: 9781118501399

86. Regalado, V., & Álvarez, A. (2020). Characterization of temperature and humidity index and heat stress in dairy cattle in two dairies in Mayabeque province, Cuba. *Cuban Journal of Agricultural Science*, *54*(1), 11-18. Available: http://scielo.sld.cu/scielo.php?script=sci_arttext&pid=S2079-34802020000100011

87. Risco, C., *et al.* (2009). Comparison of reproductive performance in lactating dairy cows bred by natural service or timed artificial insemination. *Journal of Dairy Science*, 92, 5456-5466. https://doi.org/10.3168/jds.2009-2197

88. Ríos, Á., & Villagómez, E. (2020). Reproductive analysis of Brown Swiss x Zebu and Simmental x Zebu cows under tropical conditions. *Revista MVZ Córdoba*, *25*(1), 16-23. https://doi.org/10.21897/rmvz.1637

89. Riveros, A., *et al.* (2018). Comparison of two fixed-time artificial insemination protocols in Brahman cows. *Revista MVZ Cordoba*, *23*(s), 7025-7034. https://doi.org/10.21897/rmvz.1425

90. Ronchi , B., *et al.* (2001). Influence of heat stress and feed restriction on plasma progesterone, estradiol-17β LH, FSH, prolactin and cortisol in Holstein heifers. *Livesock Production Science*, 68, 231-241. https://doi.org/10.1016/S0301-6226(00)00232-3.

91. Rodriguez, E. (2021). The importance of nutrition in reproductive efficiency of suckler cows. *Livestock*, (133), 28-29.

92. Rhoads, R., et al. (2013). Nutritional interventions to alleviate the negative consequences of heat stress. *Advances in Nutrition*, 4(3), 267-276. https://doi.org/10.3945%2Fan.112.003376

93. Rojas, C., *et al.* (2021). Background and perspectives of some priority diseases affecting bovine livestock in Mexico. *Revista Mexicana de Ciencias Pecuarias*, *12*, 111-148. https://doi.org/10.22319/rmcp.v12s3.5848

94. Romo, A., *et al.* (2019). Behavioral response of beef cattle producers in intensive finishing in hot desert climate. *Abanico Veterinario*, 9.

https://doi.org/10.21929/abavet2019.928.
https://doi.org/10.21929/abavet2019.928

95. SAS (2004). User's guide. *SAS Institute Inc., Cary, North Carolina, USA.*
96. Saumande, J., & Humblot, P. (2005). The variability in the interval between estrus and ovulation in cattle and its determinants. *Animal Reproduction Science,* 85(3-4), 171-182. https://doi.org/10.1016/j.anireprosci.2003.09.009
97. Severino, V., *et al.* (2021). Socioeconomic and technological characterization of productive systems with Criollo cattle in Campeche, Mexico. *Acta universitaria*, 31. https://doi.org/10.15174/au.2021.3102
98. Sheldon, I.M. et al. (2006). Defining postpartum uterine disease in cattle. *Theriogenology*, 65, 1516-1530. https://doi.org/10.1016/j.theriogenology.2005.08.021
99. Shipka, M., & Ellis, L. (1999). Effects of bull exposure on postpartum ovarian activity of dairy cows. *Animal Reproduction Science*, 54 (4), 237-244. https://doi.org/10.1016/s0378-4320(98)00160-2.
100. SIAP (Servicio de Información Agroalimentaria y Pesquera) (2018). "Livestock Production Statistics for Mexico". Retrieved from https://www.gob.mx/siap/acciones-y-programas/produccion-pecuaria.
101. Sice, M., *et al.* (2022). Present and future of gestation diagnosis in cattle. *Anales de Veterinaria de Murcia, 36.* Available: https://dialnet.unirioja.es/servlet/articulo?codigo=8762003
102. St-Pierre, N.R. *et al.* (2013). Economic losses from heat stress by US livestock industries. *Journal of Animal Science*, 86, E52-E77. https://doi.org/10.3168/jds.S0022-0302(03)74040-5.
103. Tapia, M., & Hepp, C. (2020). Beef cattle: maternal efficiency in breeding herds. *Instituto de Investigaciones Agropecuarias Informativo, 55.* Available: https://biblioteca.inia.cl/bitstream/handle/20.500.14001/4044/Informativo%20INIA%20N%C2%B0%2055?sequence=1
104. Thatcher, W.W., *et al.* (1994). Embryo health and mortality in sheep and cattle. *Journal of Animal Science*, 72, 16-30. https://doi.org/10.2527/1994.72suppl_316x
105. Thompson, J., *et al.* (1996). Management of summer infertility in Texas Holstein dairy cattle. *Theriogenology*, 46, 547-58. https://doi.org/10.1016/0093-691x(96)00176-8.

106. Torres, A.V.F., *et al.* (2022). Economic evaluation of reproductive and productive efficiency in productive systems with Criollo cattle in Campeche, *Mexico. Acta Universitaria*, 32, 1-15. https://doi.org/10.15174/au.2022.3501

107. Ulvshammar K. (2014). Effects of shade on milk production in Swedish dairy cows on pasture. Available: https://stud.epsilon.slu.se/6604/7/ulvshammar_k_140416.pdf.

108. Utrera, Á. R., *et al.* (2007). Estimators of genetic parameters for growth traits of Mexican Charolais cattle. *Revista Mexicana de Ciencias Pecuarias*, 45(2), 121-130. Available: http://www.redalyc.org/articulo.oa?id=61345201

109. Vallejo, D., et al. (2017). Ovulation synchronization in cattle using equine chorionic gonadotropin with and without restricted suckling. Journal of Veterinary Medicine, 35, 83-91. https://doi.org/10.19052/mv.4391

110. Van der Hurk, R., & Zhao, J. (2005). Formation of mammalian oocytes and their growth, differentiation and maturation within ovarian follicles. *Theriogenology*, 63, 1717- 1751. https://doi.org/10.1016/j.theriogenology.2004.08.005.

111. Verdoljak, J., *et al.* (2018). Reproduction and mortality of cattle breeds in subtropical climate of argentina. *Abanico Veterinario*, *8* (1), 28-35. https://doi.org/10.21929/abavet2018.81.2.

112. Viana J (2019). 2018 Statistics of embryo production and transfer in domestic farm animals. *Embryo Technology Newsletter*, 36(4), 8-25. Available: https://www.iets.org/Portals/0/Documents/Public/Committees/DRC/IETS_Data_Retrieval_Report_2018.pdf

113. Viñoles, C., *et al.* (2022). Advances in knowledge on Silvopastoral Systems in Uruguay. *Latin American Archives of Animal Production*, *30*(1), 43-53. Available: https://dialnet.unirioja.es/servlet/articulo?codigo=8658796

114. Wang, S., *et al.* (2020). Early pregnancy diagnoses based on physiological indexes of dairy cattle: a review. *Tropical Animal Health and Production*, 52, 2205-2212. https://doi.org/10.1007/s11250-020-02230-9.

115. Wolfenson, D., *et al.* (2000). Impaired reproduction in heat-stressed cattle: Basic and applied aspects. *Animal Reproduction Science*, 60-61, 535-47. https://doi.org/10.1016/S0378-4320(00)00102-0.

116. Wiersma (1990). Department of Agricultural Engineering. *The University of Arizona, Tucson.*

117. Younas, M., *et al.* (1993). Estrous and endocrine responses of lactating Holsteins to forced ventilation during summer. *Journal of Dairy Science*, 76(2), 430-436. https://doi.org/10.3168/jds.s0022-0302(93)77363-4

118. Zazueta, C., *et al.* (2021). Assessment of thermal comfort of beef cattle in intensive finishing in hot climate. *Revista de Investigaciones Veterinarias del Peru*, *32*(5). https://doi.org/10.15381/rivep.v32i5.19301. https://doi.org/10.15381/rivep.v32i5.19301.

119. Zemjanis, R. (1962). Diagnostic and therapeutic techniques in animal reproduction. Baltimore, *MD: The William and Wilikins Company.*

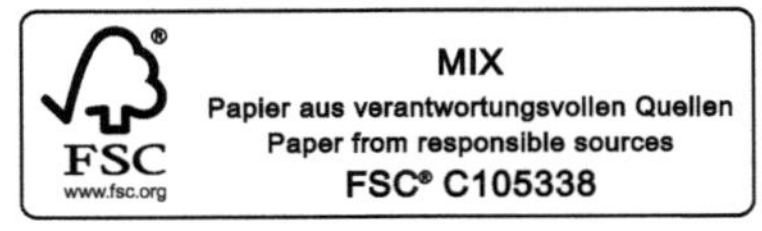

Printed by Books on Demand GmbH, Norderstedt / Germany